THE
GHOST
IN MY
BRAIN

THE
GHOST
IN MY
BRAIN

How a Concussion Stole My Life and How the
New Science of Brain Plasticity Helped Me Get It Back

CLARK ELLIOTT, PH.D.

VIKING

VIKING
Published by the Penguin Publishing Group
Penguin Random House LLC
375 Hudson Street
New York, New York 10014

USA | Canada | UK | Ireland | Australia | New Zealand | India | South Africa | China
penguin.com
A Penguin Random House Company

First published by Viking Penguin, an imprint of Penguin Publishing Group, a division of
Penguin Random House LLC, 2015

Figures and drawings by Donalee Markus

ISBN 978-0-525-42656-1

Printed in the United States of America
1   3   5   7   9   10   8   6   4   2

Set in Janson Text
Designed by Spring Hoteling

To the millions who suffer head injuries each year. There is hope.

CONTENTS

CONTENTS

PART FOUR
THE SCIENCE OF BRAIN PLASTICITY | 225

EPILOGUE | 295

FOREWORD

BY DONALEE MARKUS, PH.D.

Clark Elliott was a mystery to me when we first met. Observing him through my glass front door, I saw that it took him two minutes just to find the doorknob with his hand. When I gave him the simplest of my assessment tests—copying a geometric line drawing—his body went into bizarre contortions as he struggled to complete it. It hurt me to watch this brilliant man put so much effort into such a trivial task. In my decades-long practice in clinically applied neuroscience (CAN), this case was striking. During the two-hour evaluation session, I kept asking myself, "What could have happened in the car accident eight years ago that all of these top medical doctors have missed?" In thinking over my plan for rewiring his brain, I realized that most of Clark's cognitive and motor behaviors were likely tied to stress on his visual systems, and I wanted him to work in parallel with my highly esteemed colleague the optometrist Deborah Zelinsky, whom he went to see the following week.

Clark was an ideal client. He understood the complexity of the brain and the relationship between sensory input and behavior. And he was compliant, faithfully completing the rigorous cognitive exercises that I created for him—the brain puzzles he was to solve on a daily basis. Most important, he carefully documented his behavioral changes so that I could move him quickly through the exercises that would allow him to regain control of his personal and professional life.

Clark's story is remarkable. Through his scrupulously documented recovery, he gives a voice and provides hope to millions of people, referred to as the *walking wounded*, with mild to moderate traumatic brain injury. The plasticity of the human brain is both its power and its weakness. Although the life-sustaining parts of the human brain are "hardwired," the cognitive parts (located in the neocortex) are not. The part of the brain that allows people to think, to plan, to hope, to dream, to understand language and math, and to recognize themselves and others, is highly malleable.

This plasticity allows people to change their minds and to control their behavior, but it is also this part that suffers the greatest loss from brain injury. Much to the frustration of doctors and patients alike, cellular damage is microscopic and may be diffuse throughout the brain so that conventional scanning technologies cannot detect it.

By the time high-functioning individuals with post-traumatic head injury notice that their memories are not what they used to be, or that they have difficulty thinking through a problem they could once have easily solved, massive brain damage has occurred on a microscopic level. Because their symptoms are medically unverifiable and therefore untreatable, they are usually dismissed as the walking wounded, destined to suffer the pain, frustration, and humiliation of not knowing how much longer their condition will last or how much worse it will become. The *Designs for Strong Minds* system I have developed to treat such clients who come to me is a program based on a neurocognitive model that relies on the brain's plastic, reconfigurable nature, and uses *attention, intention,* and *rehearsal* to implement learning and behavioral change.

It is important to give credit to two individuals who contributed to Clark's cognitive restructuring success. Professor Reuven Feuerstein in 1981 introduced me to the original theoretical framework and the system that are the basis of my work, where the tools are *context-free visual puzzles* organized by logical structure, and the technique is *mediation,* to change the structure of the brain. It is from Professor Feuerstein that I learned "Intelligence is plastic. . . . Cognition is modifiable at any age." And Christine Williams of NASA provided me with the opportunity to work with our top scientists, engineers, physicists—literally our rocket scientists—from 1998 to 2005. The tools, more than three thousand paper-and-pencil instruments that I created for NASA (joined by almost ten thousand instruments for children), became the framework, the structure, and the workbooks for Clark to regain his high-level cognitive functioning skills.

Warm regards,
Donalee Markus
www.designsforstrongminds.com

FOREWORD

BY DEBORAH ZELINSKY, O.D.

After a car accident disrupted his brain function, Clark Elliott embarked on a long and difficult journey to regain mental and physical capacities. His recovery testifies to his own determination, and also to new therapeutic techniques developed by Dr. Markus and myself. At one level, Clark's story stands out because of his tenacity in pushing through successive phases of recuperation. At another, it supports the concept that visual inputs can affect brain function, which in turn can promote better coordination between brain and body systems. This theme that eyeglasses and mental activity can alter brain function, and brain function alters body function, remains at the forefront during the entire book and is very eye-opening to read.

Central eyesight, which allows us to "see" an object, is the last and slowest visual pathway to be activated during processing and yet, mistakenly, the most common way of evaluating visual function. Other pathways include peripheral eyesight that allows the brain to set a context for such objects, and many non-image-forming retinal pathways that link the external environment to internal systems that control sentience and metabolism. This last group of pathways is routed beneath conscious awareness directly from the retina to the body and affects such critical systems as balance, posture, hormones, neurotransmitters, circadian rhythms, etc. The interaction of all the non-image-forming signaling pathways modulates peripheral eyesight, and in turn the efficiency of central eyesight. Brain trauma such as that which Clark suffered often wreaks havoc on the balance of these three main visual systems.

My work in the field of neuro-optometric rehabilitation is based on the original ideas of Harry Riley Spitler and A. M. Skeffington, in the 1920s and '30s respectively. Spitler observed that specific color frequencies affected body function, and Skeffington noted that some people could see targets clearly, yet remained visually uncomfortable, often rejecting glasses and preferring to have blurry eyesight. This line of thinking that the eye has connections with both the body and the mind was advanced further by notable optometric contributors including Gerald Getman, who identified links between visual processing and motor development, and Harry Wachs, who used Piaget's concepts to link academic development in the mind with motor stimulation of the body. In the 1980s, optometrists Bruce Wolff and John Thomas used the image of an eye being one of many doorways into brain function, having entrances and exits to synchronized, multisensory processing. In the 1990s my mentor, Albert A. Sutton, taught me never to think of the eye in isolation. A decade later, Selwyn Super's fascinating book on the differences between intention, attention, and inattention helped me to solidify rehabilitative concepts. As of 2014, more than 125 European doctors are expanding their thinking to include eye/ear interactions that can be affected by glasses, based on the ideas behind my patented Z-Bell™ diagnostic system.*

One outgrowth of these decades of clinical research has been the intentional use of therapeutic glasses to break old neurological habits, allowing new habits to develop beneath conscious awareness. Neuro-optometric rehabilitation, using customized lenses, can often help patients with different kinds of injuries recover from such lingering symptoms as difficulties with balance, motor control, seizure activity, and executive functioning. Thousands of articles on retinal circuitry—linking modern neuroscience with optometry—describe the pervasive integration of brain and body systems. At the heart of neuro-optometric rehabilitation is how such research can improve the lives of patients. Babak Kateb, M.D., another visionary, founded the World Brain Mapping Association based on the interdisciplinary concepts of translational medicine. At the association's international meeting this year, neuro-optometry will be one of the featured tracks, because contemporary retinal research has clearly demonstrated how optometry can profoundly affect brain and body functions.

---

*With academic and professional titles: Harry Riley Spitler, D.O.S., M.D., Ph.D.; A. M. Skeffington, O.D., D.O.S., F.A.A.O.; Gerald Getman, O.D., D.O.S., Sc.D.; Harry Wachs, O.D.; Bruce Wolff, O.D.; John Thomas, O.D.; Albert A. Sutton, O.D., M.S., F.C.O.V.D.; Selwyn Super, D. Optom., D.Ed.; Babak Kateb, M.D., Ph.D.

Abbreviation key: O.D., D. Optom. (Doctor of Optometry); D.O.S. (Doctor of Optometric Science); Sc.D. (Doctor of Science); F.A.A.O. (Fellow, American Academy of Optometry); F.C.O.V.D (Fellow, College of Optometrists in Visual Development); D.Ed. (Doctor of Education); F.N.O.R.A. (Fellow, Neuro-Optometric Rehabilitation Association).

Clark's amazing saga was written on the basis of his meticulous notes from the moment of his brain trauma until his remarkable recovery almost a decade later. He documents not only the intricate balance between visual/spatial processing and cognition that makes us human, but also the arduous passage from one stage of recuperation to another. As readers follow his story, it is hoped that they will gain a greater understanding of how the mind-eye connection is much more than meets the eye, and how people with many types of brain problems can be helped by carefully prescribed, nontraditional eyeglasses.

Deborah Zelinsky
www.mindeyeconnection.com

AUTHOR'S NOTE

Why I Wrote This Book

This book is intended for those who have suffered from a brain injury and know it, for those who have suffered a brain injury and will not know it until they recognize aspects of their lives in these pages, for those who have family members or friends who have suffered a brain injury, and for those who are simply interested in the magnificent inner workings of the most powerful computing device on earth: the human brain.

Stories of my fellow concussion survivors have flooded the media in recent years: returning combat veterans who have suffered traumatic brain injury (TBI), professional athletes who are demanding accountability from sports leagues and helmet makers, and some of our country's youth who have suffered troubling sports concussions. Given the *millions* of TBIs that are even reported each year in the United States alone, this is, yes, a quiet plague of epidemic proportions. Yet our society is only grudgingly coming to recognize that concussions are serious and life-changing injuries that may have lingering, undiagnosed symptoms such as emotional difficulties, fatigue, learning problems, and social problems that can last a lifetime.

In my experience, the medical community's standard of care for certain classes of TBIs has not yet caught up with effective new treatments that are available. There are many excellent physicians who have been exposed to current research in "brain plasticity" (wherein parts of the brain can be trained to compensate for other, injured parts), especially those physicians working with sports and military head injuries. However, it is unfortunately true that many M.D.s, including leading neurologists—as well as putative leading rehabilitation institutions—are as of the time of this writing unwittingly out of date when it comes to accurately diagnosing and treating concussion. This is unspeakably sad for those who are needlessly suffering and believe they have nowhere to turn.

The later chapters of this book that cover the science behind my recovery may also be highly revealing for those who suspect that they suffer from some form of attention difficulty, such as ADD, or suspect that a family member does. In the process of my recovery I realized that many of the features of such attention difficulties significantly overlap with those manifesting as concussion symptoms. From the many anecdotes I've heard from my university students, and others, I think we should be highly suspicious that some of these attention difficulties are rooted in prior, sometimes even mild, head injuries. How many times have I heard, "Oh, yes—now that you ask, I did start having this trouble last year after I had that [car accident / skiing mishap / skateboard fall / soccer concussion]. . . ."

The small changes that can occur in one's brain from even a quite forgettable bump on the head can masquerade in subtle ways such as personality oddities, trouble with multitasking, sleep disturbances, and even just growing old. Who would have thought to consider that slip on an icy doorstep five years ago as the culprit behind having a slight sense of being out of sync at unpredictable times, or having trouble managing appointments?

As a professor of artificial intelligence and cognitive science, I have shared some of the concepts covered in this book about how brains work with my classes, including the ideas behind several leading-edge cognitive restructuring, and neuro-optometric, treatments. It has been striking that I have never failed to have, in each such course, at least two students talk to me after class about their extreme interest in the material because of their own information-processing difficulties. This suggests to me that the kinds of brain difficulties experienced by *concussives* (as in, those who have suffered concussions)—albeit in much milder forms than my own—are far more widespread than we might traditionally suspect, especially among high-functioning, intelligent people who are very good at masking such problems.

One of the things concussives share is the feeling of having become an alien being. We still walk and talk and act as though we are part of the human race, but it doesn't feel that way inside. Essential parts of our brains that convey what it means to be fully human have disappeared—vanished in that moment of impact when we tripped on the stairs, or crashed into an arena wall. Instead there is a strange feeling of nostalgia, a longing for who we used to be.

Normals—those who haven't suffered from concussions—will take for granted the countless small operations their brains perform as they think and gracefully move their bodies through the day. But a concussive loses the ability to manage the staggering complexity of the systems that implement these operations, and as a result loses not only basic cognitive and motor functions, but also a larger sense of self-identity, and identity in relation to the world. This makes us odd beasts—a cross between what amputees may experience with phantom limb syndrome, and what *hemispatial neglect* patients have when they suddenly lose half of their world: On the one hand, with a phantom limb, amputees are constantly reminded of what they used to be, of being whole. On the other hand, neglect patients are missing part of themselves and their world, and while they feel a sense of loss, they can no longer even imagine what it is they are missing. For a long time I lived in such a dual-natured limbo.

This book captures my harrowing yet ultimately fascinating odyssey as a concussive. For almost a decade, and even while struggling mightily—sometimes just to get through a doorway, or down a flight of stairs—I was constantly observing, analyzing, and recording the events unfolding in my life, and the ways in which my damaged brain was trying to make sense of them. I took twelve hundred pages of notes, and through them I became the subject of my own long-range experiment in cognition—exploring the relationship between mind and body, and the inner mind and outer world. Along the way I learned a great deal about how the *healthy* human brain works as well—leaving me in awe of this sublime and formidable computational device.

The book's title is a play on the phrase *the Ghost in the*

Machine—and thus an indirect allusion to the seminal French philosopher René Descartes's idea of a mind-body dualism. Descartes believed these two agencies were separate—that the mind existed separate from the body. Oxford philosopher Gilbert Ryle disagreed, and in 1949 used the phrase to poke fun at Cartesian dualism. Although the jury is still out on this question, I know from personal experience—such as on a snowy night we'll soon see in downtown Chicago—that the mind and body are intricately intertwined. But the meaning of the title goes beyond this duality. Readers will come to understand that the ghost in my book is the sense of my true self—the "me" that was sent into exile in the moment of a car crash. Years later I underwent cognitive treatment based on the new principles of brain plasticity. Shortly thereafter, one evening outside my office at DePaul University, I felt the ghost return. My old self—the ghost of who I had been and who I so longed to be once more—had come back. I wept tears of joy that I was no longer sentenced to life as an alien living among real humans.

Above all, this is an illustrated tour through the odd, awe-inspiring, painful, scary, tragic, and fascinating world of brain injury, but one that in this case has the all-too-rare happy ending—an ending that is yet also likely to be possible for many thousands of those still exclusively locked into more traditional treatments (or nontreatments, as the case may be) for concussion.

As recently as four years ago I was told by local experts in the Chicago medical community that the only course of action I could take to deal with my symptoms was to learn to live with them. This would have entailed giving up my tenured position as a university professor, retiring into poverty from all forms of work, giving up the custodianship of my children, and perhaps becoming a ward of the state.

And yet today, through the courageous work of two brilliant Chicago-area researcher-clinicians, each of whom works at the leading edge of brain science relative to certain kinds of traumatic brain injury, I am almost without symptoms. The efforts of Donalee Markus, Ph.D., who rebuilds brains by using puzzles, and of Deborah Zelinsky, O.D., who accesses the visual cortex and regrows brain pathways using prescription eyeglasses, gave me back my life.

This is my story.

PART ONE
CONCUSSION

MIDNIGHT

Just before nine o'clock, on a frigid night in early 2002, I completed my three-hour lecture on artificial intelligence at DePaul University's downtown campus. I was exhausted, and ready to head for home, but it took me another two hours to make my way to the sixth floor of the building across the street, then crawl down the hall to my office and there rest in the dark and the quiet until I was able to attempt my journey north to Evanston. Finally, at eleven, I left the building again and headed off through the brutal wind, intending to walk the five blocks to my car, parked near the lake on Columbus Drive.

Two and a half years earlier I had been rear-ended while waiting at a stoplight in nearby Morton Grove. It had been a relatively minor accident, but it had left me with brain damage from a concussion. Because of it, I found the scene now unfolding to be quite common: sitting behind the podium in my classroom until long after the students had left, surreptitiously crawling down the hallways when I could no longer walk, then later lying on the floor of my office doing absolutely nothing until I lost track of time. And now I had to face a bizarre gauntlet that would take me across nearby Grant Park to my car, before making the long drive home.

It was scary cold over by the lake at this late hour, but I thought: *I can make it.*

I was walking reasonably well—but quite slowly—when I left my building on Wabash next to the El tracks. As I rounded the first corner at Jackson Boulevard, snow flurries began swirling around my head, flickering in the streetlights. Cars carrying late-working professionals raced down the street next to me as they too headed for home. I started having trouble navigating through the visual chaos around me, and I began to lose my balance when the wind gusted around the corners of the skyscrapers. I shied away from the traffic, and reached out to hold on to the sides of the buildings as I walked. By the time I had gone only two short blocks my brain was already beginning to tire again from the effort.

I stopped to rest on the corner before crossing through the late Michigan Avenue traffic. But even then I only made it to the center island before having to pause for several more traffic-light cycles. I thought, *This is going to be tricky*, and considered turning back. But turning back would mean forming another plan for how to get home, or perhaps where to sleep, and I couldn't manage it. *Easier to go on*, I thought. *It's just across the park.*

By the next block, as I crossed over the Illinois Central tracks and headed up the slight incline, I was moving ever . . . more . . . slowly. I finally made it to the edge of the snow-encrusted park, and started diagonally across it toward my parking spot on the other side. I was by now shuffling along with a strange, slightly pigeon-toed gait and only managing a few inches with each step. My jaw hung down, and my head bobbed from side to side as I moved.

I felt the onset of a visual impairment similar to what cinematographers call the "Dolly Zoom Effect," famously used in the opening rooftop chase of Hitchcock's *Vertigo*: Jimmy Stewart is hanging from a rain gutter about to plunge to his death. As he looks down into the alley below, the background visual scene bends and the alley floor drops away, even though the foreground stays the same size. This was the scene playing out in front of me now, except in real life, and I couldn't stop it. With each step I took forward, the distant goal toward which I was walking appeared two steps farther away.

Despite the frightening challenges such breakdowns engendered, I often perversely experienced a kind of existential wonder during these episodes as well, as I watched the great machine disintegrating before my eyes. I became a rare observer of the fascinating structures from which the unfiltered world was actually formed. Simple relationships all around me deteriorated into an unfolding chaos of increasingly eccentric patterns. Time morphed into something hypnotically strange and disjoint. It was all spooky geometry linking one frozen moment to the next.

From within this dim labyrinth I was still just barely managing to power the engine of thought. As I progressed across the park, I had to carefully map out the *shape* of each step from within the shadowy white images, and force my legs to follow the path these shapes described: *left foot forward . . . right foot forward . . .* But my world was growing increasingly fragmented, and as I lost my ability to put the elusive fragments together to form visual goals, I simultaneously lost the ability to walk.

After *forty minutes*—three quarters of the way to my car but still less than four blocks from where I had started—I stopped moving altogether. My brain resources were used up. No crafty logic, no amount of physical strength, and not even an abundance of raw will could bridge the gap between my intention and my feet.

I had known the risks of getting stuck in the park when I went to work in the early afternoon, but I made my decisions from the most deeply felt sense of obligation. Not only did I love my work at the university, but keeping my job was not negotiable: ten people lived on my salary, including what would soon be five children. What other real choice did I have but to run the various gauntlets when I had to, including this one tonight? So now, once again, here I was. From long experience I knew there was not much for me to do but simply wait to find out how this particular scene in my life was going to end.

At this point my world had collapsed inward on itself: the concepts of *distance* and *left and right* had become dim memories. Every discrete event, independent of all context, slowly emerged from the ether and then receded into the void. My sensory filters had deserted me too, and within the great arc that was left I didn't even know where my body ended and the rest of the world began.

So now what? Despite the circumstances I was still at least the shell of a professor who worked at building artificial brains. It was my job to solve hard problems. I looked down at my feet and shouted at myself to walk, but I knew it was hopeless. I had lost the mysterious *initiative* that impels us all forward when we walk, and I knew that without brain rest I wouldn't be getting it back. I considered lying down in the snow—which would at least give my damaged vestibular system a rest—but because of the bitter cold it seemed unwise. I might never get up again.

In the end I just stood there staring into the distance, absolutely still: slowly and painfully freezing, my jaw hanging slack, my arms out to the side for balance, doing nothing at all. I was seeking a special kind of visual peace, a calming of the outward landscape that would give my brain the cognitive rest it needed. But I had to be careful not to slide into a meditative state—because meditation would require attention and the ability to sense some mystical structure in the nothingness. Each of these would require the forming of spatial images and further deplete the scant brain resources I had left. What I needed instead was a completely different kind of nothing: a run-of-the-mill, down-to-earth, completely, utterly boring nothing of the kind that tortures schoolchildren at 2:30 in the afternoon on beautiful warm days in June.

Midnight was approaching, and I started to shiver uncontrollably. After another twenty minutes—*an hour since leaving my office*—I had the vague thought that perhaps this was finally the end; I would become just another statistic of exposure, lost to the cruel Chicago winter. I reflected with some resignation—an internal shrugging of my shoulders—that this was going to be a lonely way to die, alone in the wind and the cold like this, unable to move. I felt ashamed of my helplessness—all I needed to do was start walking. But there was nothing I could do.

Because of a neurological quirk, I was holding my hands in an odd position, forefingers and thumbs sticking up and outward to form an "L," while my other fingers bent downward—apparently some elemental effort to help me keep my balance.

With conscious effort I clenched my hands into fists inside my padded leather gloves to keep them warm. But going against my primal neural programming in even this minor way drained me of the last effort I could muster. My system was shutting down.

Be brilliant, Clark, and come up with a solution. But don't you dare use your brain—save every last mental resource to connect your body to the visual goal up ahead, and move your feet toward it. I wished for some magical solution that would float up out of the ether of my subconscious, one that I could conceive of without having to think at all. But I didn't know how to make this happen.

I was so tired—so bone-deep achingly tired. And somewhere in the cauldron of forbidden thoughts that I could not allow to form, I was also tired of being so tired—just like this— all the time, of having to struggle each day to perform the simplest of actions. But this was not a matter of emotional distress—most days my natural disposition was still upbeat, and I was often simply a careful observer, curious about what my obviously changed future would bring. My global fatigue was, instead, a deep exhaustion from the *physical* grind of thinking, and the resulting constant pain.

After a while an overwhelming desire came over me to lie down in the soft white blanket of snow covering the grass in front of me. The irony was that even though I was aware of the risk of dying, I was by this time no longer able to see what this meant. I couldn't conceive of it—something about time, something about calendars, something about endings, and the right-hand side of a timeline ending in nothing. The difference between life and death had lost its structure in the same way the line between my inner self and the world around me had vanished.

It was too much, too hard, too fuzzy to try to understand. I just wanted to curl up with my back to the stinging wind, and disappear.

But in another twist of irony, *I didn't know how to lie down.* I couldn't see the relationships between the vertical and horizontal planes around me, or how my body fit into them either. My concussed brain couldn't make sense of motion, and the sequence of motion over time. It didn't "get" any of this in the geometric way that would have allowed me to move. Without *seeing*, I couldn't initiate, and without initiating I couldn't lie down in the snow to die. . . .

THE SIZE OF THE PROBLEM: THE MAGNIFICENCE OF THE HUMAN BRAIN

The human brain is a magnificent device, and the complexity of the human mind it supports is staggering to ponder. It is not possible for us fully to understand the enormity of the changes that take place when someone suffers a traumatic brain injury (TBI)—a concussion*—without first having some idea of the phenomenal (astronomical!) computational powers of the device we are considering.

Some supercomputer researchers estimate they'll need

---

*There is a lot of confusion, if not outright controversy, about the differences between traumatic brain injury (TBI), mild traumatic brain injury (mTBI/MTBI), post-concussion syndrome (PCS), and other labels, relative to how persistent the symptoms are: initial unconsciousness, score on the Glasgow Coma Scale, etc. There is also much that is outright wrong about measures of the persistence of symptoms. I will use the simplest definition of TBI—a physical trauma to the head causing brain injury—and concussion mostly interchangeably as terms in this nonmedical, nonlegal text.

exaflop computing speeds (1,000,000,000,000,000,000 floating-point operations a second) to model a single human brain. Put in layman's terms, that's 50 *million* desktop computers all networked together—and a single such modern desktop is a pretty powerful device, far more sophisticated than the big boxes of the 1960s and '70s that might each support a company with thousands of employees. Another way to picture this is that 50 million desktop computers laid end-to-end would stretch halfway around the earth, with another three thousand miles to spare.

For those of us who are trying to mimic some of the brain's systems, these are not even the impressive numbers. Rather it is the *design* of the system—the organization of the software, so to speak, and the impregnated information—that is the truly extraordinary aspect of who we are.

Imagine for a second that you are back standing outside the front door of the place you lived when you were five years old. What color is the door? Does it have glass in it? Does it open outward or inward? Are there steps in front? A landing? Is there a doorknob or a latch? On which side are the hinges? Remember that door?

Estimates on the size of human memory vary widely. We are not even sure how to define it because, for example, retrieving information from memory also modifies it at the same time. But by almost all reckoning, it is very, very, large.

To get a handle on the numbers, let's imagine that we are writing everything we remember down on sheets of paper, in a 12-point font, on both sides of the paper (one byte per character). The more we have to remember, the more pieces of paper we put on our stack. The size of our memory is the height of the stack of paper. So how tall is the stack?

Harvard researchers have been able to store large amounts of information in DNA molecules, and if our brain were made of pure DNA, our memory-capacity stack of paper might stretch out into space for 2,485,795,454 miles—or circle the earth 100 million times. So we know that biological systems can store a great deal of information! Many estimates of actual human memory capacity have the pile of paper extending a much humbler distance—merely up to the moon and back.

But now we ask about the real magic—how did you get 238,000 miles up to the moon alongside that stack of paper, halfway back, another six hundred miles, twelve hundred feet, eight inches, fifty-eight pages, and two paragraphs along to find the exact location of the information about that front door you haven't seen in twenty years? How did you know to look there? How did you do that in less than a second? Because that is typically how long it takes us to retrieve that long-disused information . . .

What holds us in the greatest awe is not merely the hardware, but rather the design of the truly elegant system that runs on it, giving us the human mind.

And when we start talking about our *minds*—that which really makes us human—the numbers get even more staggering. At the University of Leicester, James Nelms, Declan Roberts, Suzanne Thomas, and David Starkey calculated that capturing everything that could contribute to a human's mental state would require 2.6 tredecillion bits (2.6 followed by 42 zeros).* In their fun paper, they note that to transmit that much information using a *Star Trek*–like teleporter, but at

---

* "P4_4 Travelling by Teleportation," *Journal of Physics Special Topics*, November 6, 2012, https://physics.le.ac.uk/journals/index.php/pst/article/view/558/380.

high-speed Internet bit rates, it would take . . . several hundred thousand times the current age of the universe.

To simulate concussion damage to a human brain then, we'll need to gather together those 50 million desktop computers, the 500,000-mile-high stack of paper, and the almost inconceivable amount of information it takes to construct a human *mind*, then loose a hurricane on the system, ripping out network lines, laying waste to vast sections of memory, and sending landslides to smash hundreds of thousands of computers.

In this way we can imagine the size of the problem we are trying to address: with a single blow to the head—in that moment of impact from concussion—we've caused staggering losses in computational power to the unimaginably complex systems that go such a long way in making us human.

Fortunately, this magnificent device is also largely plastic and able to reconfigure itself over time, borrowing a little here, and a little there, and in this way able to restore much of its lost functioning—though, as we will see, not always without a little clever jump-starting of the stalled processes.

THROUGH THE KALEIDOSCOPE

. . . My time was running out, but I was still stuck in the middle of Grant Park. And now, not only was my brain fatigued, but my mind was also growing dull from the onset of hypothermia. My body was giving up. I could not feel my toes or my fingers. I was fading away.

The question was, *How do I get moving before it is too late?*

Then magic happened. I swayed in the wind and tipped forward. My left foot moved on its own to keep me from falling, then my right foot, then my left again. *Stump, stump, stump.* I stared intently at the now inconceivably distant horizon where I knew my car was. *There is where I am going.* My jaw dropped farther, and my tongue hung down in my mouth. I could not feel the soles of my frozen feet. My index fingers popped out again, to help with balance, and I walked with a bent-kneed, shuffling gait—like a zombie. I willed myself toward my car a few inches at a time.

Within each unfolding moment, my world was made of fractured images: little scenes of blades of grass poking through the snow, of darkened tree branches, lights in the distance, and night shadows. Nothing was whole. The Dolly Zoom Effect was in full force, and though I knew, intuitively, that my car was just up ahead—thirty feet away—it still *looked* an impossible half mile distant. My feet were again coming . . . *to* . . . *a* . . . *stop*. . . . Out of desperation I changed tactics, and just *reached* for the car, let my feet walk toward the *feeling* of it, almost within my grasp. And then at last, from within the chaotic tunnel of my senses, my long journey—the first stage in the gauntlet—was finally over.

Now began the second stage. I still had to unlock the door, get in, and turn the car on. But I couldn't work it. I'd lost the concept of *center*. I had no internal representation, or visual understanding of *circle, target, middle, inside*. . . . Without these concepts I couldn't get my hand to move toward the lock, or put the key in the slot.

This situation may be a little difficult for nonconcussives—"normals"—to comprehend. There was nothing wrong with my eyes themselves, and I knew what I had to do: *put the key in the lock, open the door.* The problem was that I could not spatially or cognitively conceive of the *shape* of the problem. I stared at the door, the lock, my hand, the keys in my hand, wanting to get the door open but unable to form a physical plan to achieve my goal. I even knew the concept of *center* was still somewhere in my brain—I could feel it—but I just couldn't access it. I thought, *If I can't unlock the door, I'm going to have to walk back to my office and try again later.* I shuffled around to the front of the car and slipped down onto the frozen slush in the street, with my back against the car's front bumper. I knew I couldn't make it back to my office. I had no plan at all. No voice spoke. No thought came to me for a long time.

Then, from within the kaleidoscope, the magic rose up one last time. I pulled my stiff and cramping body to my feet. With a final extreme effort, my eyes saucer-wide and three inches from the door lock, my right hand waving around in random circles as though with no direction at all, I finally found the lock, pushed my key in, and opened the door.

I had passed through the second stage of the gauntlet.

Now came the third: maneuvering my body through the doorway in the side of the car. But once again, I couldn't *see* it. I couldn't make sense of the opening through which I was to pass. I pleaded with myself: *Get in the car, you idiot. Don't think about it—just get in and sit down.* But I couldn't do it. Instead I stood there staring off into the void, as I felt myself falling into the tunnel that reached out before me. My eyes grew wide with the effort.

Yet over time I'd developed strategies to compensate for doorways. When I couldn't propel myself in the usual way, I'd learned to spin, and dance myself through them. But now, in addition to not being able to *see* the opening, I could no longer *turn right* either. The right side of my world just tapered off into oblivion. So instead, I turned left, away from the door and away from the seat—all the way around in a full circle. I turned once, then again, and then again after that, using a strange-looking, index-fingers-out, head-turned-sideways, half-swinging motion. At last I was able to weave and bob myself into the car.

Thankfully, getting the key in the ignition was easier, and

within five minutes I had the engine running. I glanced at the clock on the dashboard. *Twelve-thirty*. It had taken me an hour and a half to make the five-block trip from my office.

I rested with the car idling until 2:00 A.M., staring at a tree in the park, completely still, completely exhausted, unaccountably hungry, but warm. A tricky moment came and went, as a suspicious cop came by, opened his window, and demanded to know why I was sitting there idling the engine. But in the end it was too cold to get out of his car, so after "rousting" me in this way, he drove away.

Soon after, sufficiently recovered, I headed for home. I never drove my car when I was under cognitive duress. But as long as my brain was sufficiently rested when I started out, then I would be okay to drive. In fact, if I was not too debilitated when I set out, the act of driving was itself restorative. Something about the staring straight ahead, and the regular motion along the sides of the road from the vanishing point past the periphery of my eyes, helped ease my impairment. Understanding directions could be tricky, as could making driving decisions, but on this night I was mindlessly following a well-worn path home, and I made the trip in about thirty minutes, without incident.

I had passed through the fourth stage of the gauntlet—but I was not done yet.

It took me another hour to get into my house from my car, though I was parked only forty feet from my front door. Finally, at 3:30 A.M., I dropped my belongings on the floor, removed my shoes, climbed the stairs to my bedroom, and lay down on my bed. In this state, sleep was still not possible. I knew that the visual processing required for dreaming would overload me when my brain was this tired. I would get sick. So, instead of sleeping, I lay in bed staring at the ice-covered branches outside my window for another hour. Then, with my brain sufficiently recovered, seven and a half hours after my class was over, I finally let myself drift off.

Another day in my life as a concussive had come to a close.

THE CRASH

On September 27th, 1999, my world as I had known it for forty-three years ended.

I was sitting at a stoplight at the intersection of Oakton and Gross Point Road in Morton Grove, Illinois, on my way to give a lecture at one of DePaul University's suburban campuses, waiting behind two other cars. A steady drizzle was falling.

Without warning, a Jeep Cherokee skidded on the wet pavement and slammed into the back of my Mazda sedan. My head bounced off the headrest behind me, and then was flung forward. I saw stars, and blacked out for a second. I was groggy, but pulled my car out of the busy intersection, around the corner, and parked on the side of Gross Point Road. I felt shaken up, but only in the way anyone who had been in a relatively minor car crash might.

A Morton Grove police officer arrived to take the accident report, and I got out of my car to meet him.

"Get back in your car and sit there until the ambulance comes!" he said, after he got a look at me. "I'm calling them now." This was puzzling to me. I couldn't understand why he was so concerned.

At one point, while we were waiting, I went to sit in the passenger seat of the other driver's Jeep. While chatting with her about a previous accident she had had that totaled her old car, I took my driver's license out of my wallet and showed it to her. But this did not make sense, because part of me understood that *I had already shown the woman my license*—in fact, just a few minutes before. After all, this is the ordinary thing: when you show a license to someone, then you know that you have done so. In this case, I *knew* that I had shown her my license, but another part of me—the part that had prompted me to show it to her in the first place—could not get the message that the task was already completed. Thus I didn't feel certain that I had performed the task, so I asked her again—would she like to see it? And then later, once more.

This would become a common occurrence: knowing something, but not knowing that I knew it in the part of my brain that needed that information to stop—or alter—the low-level generation of speech, cognitive thought processes, and physical actions. In this way I often knew exactly what was going on, could remember it later as I now clearly remember this event from fifteen years ago, and could even describe some strange, brain-damaged process while it was happening. But this still left me helpless to alter the processes that I was observing.

The ambulance came, and a pair of young paramedics, a

small man and a large one, had me sit inside it as they examined me.

"Do you know your name?" asked the bigger one.

I thought about it. It seemed like an easy enough question. But nothing immediately came to mind. I was reaching into the usual place in my mind, and retrieving nothing at all. *How odd*, I thought. After a minute I managed, "Sure. Clark Elliott."

"Well, Mr. Elliott, I think you'd better come with us to get checked out at the hospital."

"Whoa!" I said. "I can't do that. I have to get to class."

"Listen, Mr. Elliott," said the smaller paramedic, "pardon my expression, but you're pretty fucked up here. We really need to take you to the hospital."

"Thank you for your concern," I said, smiling at him, "but I'm fine. I really can't go with you because I have to teach tonight."

I didn't hurt very much. I'd given a thousand lectures over twelve years without ever missing one. It would take a lot to make me miss class. My students were expecting me to show up shortly and teach for three hours. I felt strange, but *I could not recall what it was like to not feel strange.*

I couldn't make sense of what they wanted me to do. I couldn't *see* it in the normal way. So, I refused to go to the hospital.

"Okay," said the larger paramedic. "We can't stop you. You've got to sign these release forms, and then we'll let you go. But you are doing the wrong thing." I climbed out of the ambulance and went back to my car.

The police officer knocked on my window, signaling to roll it down. "I need your insurance card," he said. I knew the card was in my car. I sat there for a minute, then opened the glove box and took out a small pile of papers. But that was as far as I got. I stared at the papers in front of me without knowing what to do with them.

The officer didn't understand that I really did know exactly where the insurance card was—it was in my hand. And I didn't know how to explain to him that for some reason I couldn't sort it out from the five other items I had in my hand and give it to him. He got tired of waiting, and instead confiscated my license—an act that would have significant repercussions later that evening when I went to retrieve it.

The officer gave me directions to get to the police station. They were quite simple—only two turns—but to my surprise, I couldn't make sense of them. Instead, with some effort, I wrote them down. I would return after class, post a cash bond, and get my license back.

The back of my Mazda was all smashed in, but the car was still running fine. My red tail lenses were cracked, but my brake lights still worked, so I drove to work, mindlessly following the path I had taken many times before. Fortunately, although I had eight miles to go through heavy traffic, I only had to make a single left turn to get to DePaul's O'Hare campus. Later that evening I thought it odd that I could not remember even a single thing about the rest of my drive to work.

The details of my evening-class lecture are spotty. I worked on autopilot, covering the very familiar material. I lectured sitting down. There were difficult moments when I just stopped in the middle of the lecture, and I had to rest several times by putting my head down on my desk. But DePaul's graduate students are a bright, multiethnic, salt-of-the-earth sort of crowd, and we joked about my loopiness being caused by the automobile accident. None of us took it seriously.

After my lecture I couldn't get up from my chair. Oddly, I had trouble getting through the door of the classroom. Then, when I reached the single flight of stairs that led to the ground floor, I froze up. I couldn't seem to *see* the stairs, even though my eyes were working fine. My feet simply wouldn't move. After ten minutes someone helped me down the stairs, while I clutched the banister. I had trouble understanding the geometry of the revolving door.

Once outside, I became disoriented. The well-lit parking lot was now only sparsely populated. It had a straightforward, traditional layout bordering two sides of the classroom building. But even so, I couldn't find my own car in it—something that had never happened to me before. I wandered around in the lot, but had no sense of its spatial nature, or of my car's placement within the space. I couldn't make sense of *car-ness* either, and when I encountered objects as I wandered around the lot, it took me some time even to figure out that they were cars.

At some point I must have found my car, because later I was driving home in it, but I don't remember how that came about.

My goal was to stop at an ATM, withdraw cash for a bond, drive to the police station, and retrieve my driver's license. It took me twenty minutes to withdraw the cash, concentrating intensely, looking at my hands, looking at my ATM card, imagining what the digits of my PIN meant, looking at the ATM display, trying to form a plan. The problem was that I could not *see* the sequence of steps in a linear fashion, and without seeing them I could not get my arms and hands to move. I was working so hard that it never even occurred to me that I should probably not be spending so long on such a trivial operation. I did not feel the least bit confused. I knew exactly what I was doing, and in my own way was entirely coherent, methodically solving the steps of a difficult puzzle. In fact, I was hyperobservant of the raw building blocks of the reality we typically filter out, which state is the antithesis of being delusional. Yet at the same time I was in the grip of one of the dominant themes that would now become a peculiar part of my life: *I did not recognize that there was anything wrong.*

Next I had to retrieve my license from the police station, which entailed a simple trip three blocks south from Dempster Street, the main thoroughfare, to get there. But now I discovered that something else had gone missing.

All my life I had had a nearly infallible sense of the North-South-East-West grid on the surface of the earth, and my orientation within it. If I lost my sense of north for even a moment I grew uncomfortable and made it a point to become immediately reoriented. But now, for the first time, I had no idea where north was, and had completely lost my sense of the NSEW grid. As it turned out, I wouldn't find more than the slightest part of it again for eight years.

So, without understanding why it was hard for me, I drove around in circles for an hour trying to find the station, trying to understand which streets were south of Dempster, which streets ran east and west, and so on.

At this point I experienced another weird phenomenon: I was *slowing down*. It was taking me longer and longer to decide whether to turn left or turn right. I had a strange sense of my mainspring just winding down. I was not sleepy, but just getting increasingly unable to function. Yet, oddly, at the same time the voice in my head—the ongoing dialogue about who I was and what I was doing—was for the most part operating in real time, at full speed, and observing everything.

Finally, I found the police station. I don't recall the exact sequence of events, but I do remember clearly my fear that the police were growing suspicious that I was intoxicated.* Using the last of my resources, I put on a game face and explained to them that I was exhausted because I had just come from a long day at work, and that I had been in an automobile accident earlier in the day. I had a sense that my believability hung in the balance, but in the end the desk officer decided to let it pass. I left the station in a hurry, then sat in my car outside for several minutes before I recovered enough from my having to "fake normalcy," which was exhausting, to be able to negotiate my way around the corner, away from the station, park the car, and rest.

Although I was clearly having cognitive difficulties, it did not affect my native ability to drive the way, say, having had alcohol would. I most noticed impairment in the form of not knowing directions, not being sure where I wanted to go if there was a choice, and in my great fatigue. But my ability to drive, and my emergency responses, were working well enough, and my reaction time was the same as always. The best analogy to consider is that it is entirely possible to know when you are too sleepy to drive safely, and make the appropriate, safe choice not to do so.†

I finally arrived home at one o'clock in the morning, after driving for three hours, which included two hours of simply wandering around in a fog not knowing quite where I was. It

---

*That these memories are dark is significant to me now, because it would not be a common occurrence in the years to come. It appears that such "missing pieces" of my life story were a feature only of the very early days after the crash.

†Although I many times made the choice not to drive, or to rest before doing so, in the fifty thousand miles covered during this period I never got a ticket or came close to causing any kind of accident.

was hard for me to get up out of the car. It was hard for me to walk from the car to the house. I had a strange and persistent difficulty unlocking my front door.

Despite my extreme fatigue, I felt too unsettled, too *wrong* to go to sleep. So I just took off my shoes and sat in my old Eames chair to rest for a while instead. I was living alone in the gutted house I was rebuilding, so there was no one to help.

My next memory was from ten o'clock the next morning. I was physically exhausted, and still sitting in the chair. I had stayed there all night without realizing that anything was wrong.

I tried to get up and start my day. But to my chagrin, I discovered that I couldn't move. I was giving the command to my body: "Get up!" but it was not listening. It was perplexing. *What does this mean?* I asked myself. I moved my head to the left and the right without much trouble. But, when I again told myself to get up, nothing happened. Nor could I move my arms. Intuitively I knew that I was not paralyzed, but my body was simply not responding to my commands.

Finally, after a very long three minutes, once I was able to manage the smallest *initiation* of motion I was able to stand up and move normally. Over the next hour I noticed several more instances of my being unable to initiate action. I brushed any concern aside, telling myself that my muscles had just been "shaken up" more than I realized the day before in the accident, and that because the muscles were sore and tired, it was hard for me to get them to respond.

SOMETHING IS WRONG

On Wednesday morning, two days after the accident, I phoned the other driver's insurance office. As the representative spoke, I was having trouble making sense of what she was saying. I felt strangely out-of-balance and nauseated because her words were coming in through just one ear, and I couldn't seem to form mental pictures fast enough to follow her. In the end I just wrote down the firm's address, and the words "Right away. Appointment."

The short phone call left me exhausted.

"Hey, you've got to get going!" I told myself repeatedly as the morning wore on, but the best I could manage was to make lunch.

By the early afternoon, not only was I unhappy with myself for getting nothing done, but I also had a very strong sense that *something was wrong*, and had been wrong all day. But I couldn't figure out what it was, and this was getting increasingly annoying. Finally, out of frustration, I just stood in my living room, determined to get to the bottom of it. Over the course of fifteen minutes I concentrated intensely, scanning my environment for clues. The top of my head began to ache, and also the back of my neck just under my skull. I held my breath to deal with the pain. I sweated with the effort, and my body began to give out from the stress of pushing myself so hard. But finally I figured it out: I had put my shoes on the wrong feet in the morning when I had gotten up six hours earlier.

At this point, for the first time in two days, it finally occurred to me that there was something going on besides sore muscles from being "shaken up" in a car accident. It was not supposed to take me fifteen minutes to be able to figure out that I'd been wearing my shoes on the wrong feet all day, right? And yet I still didn't understand that there was anything really wrong—how could there be? I just couldn't "get" it. On the surface everything was in order.

I called the family doctor, and he said that I should go to the emergency room and get checked out—the standard response.

I thought about going to the hospital right away, instead of to the insurance claims office, but I was *unable to make a decision* about what I should do.

"This is weird!" I thought. "Just pick one." But I couldn't. After ten minutes of sitting in my chair waiting for a plan to come to me, nothing happened. In the end, without thought, I managed to focus on getting the car sorted out first. It was the fear of being without transport to get around in my busy life that finally made the decision *for* me.

I drove to the address that I'd written down. The navigation was unaccountably hard for me. My sense of time became distorted as I began to focus on minute details of the environment around me: the color of a sign, the smell of the car, smudges on the windshield, the wind blowing leaves across the road. By the time I arrived I had a terrible headache. I was looking, and feeling, distinctly disheveled after two days of managing almost nothing. I had not shaved, or changed my clothes. I sat in the car for twenty minutes, staring off into space, then went into the office and talked to the receptionist—a large, unpleasant woman who looked as though she had had to calm down irate insurance claimants all day.

"Hi," I said. "My name is Elliott. I spoke to someone this morning about my car."

"Okay," she said. "Why are you here? Do you have an appointment?"

"I'm not sure," I said slowly, hesitating between words. "One of the people you insure ran into me. I was told I have to come in right away."

"If you don't have an appointment [. . .]" I was having a lot of trouble processing her words. I couldn't follow her.

"I'm sorry," I said, "could you speak more slowly? I don't understand what you are saying."

She spoke more loudly, as though I were hard of hearing, which, because of the phonosensitivity I was experiencing from the concussion, was painful. But she did not speak more slowly. Because she was now annoyed, her consonants became increasingly percussive, which felt like small hammers rapping against my skull. I was even less well able to follow her than I was before.

The receptionist scowled at me. "Just a minute," she said, and walked back and spoke to another woman whom I took to be the *handler-of-difficult-customers* person in the office. The second woman looked something up on the computer and then came over to me.

"Mr. Elliott, you have an appointment on Friday," she said in a painfully loud voice. I winced and tried to make sense of what she was saying to me. *Friday?* I said to myself. *Friday . . .* I didn't know what that meant. I had no sense of the flow of time through the days of the week. I could see the word "Friday" in front of my eyes, but nothing else came to mind.

"Is it possible you could have someone look at my car if I was willing to wait for a spot?" I asked. "It's right outside."

"Our office [. . .]" she said loudly, glaring at me. I tried to follow, but I couldn't make out what this woman was saying, either.

"I'm . . . sorry . . . what . . . ?" I said hesitantly. I was having trouble forming my words, and was slurring them slightly.

She interrupted me in an even louder voice, speaking even more rapidly: "OUR OFFICE [. . .]" Her face was determined, and angry. I covered my ears with my hands, closing my eyes.

Once I covered my ears, she stopped altogether, clearly offended. "I am going to have to ask you to leave the premises right now," she demanded.

What was happening to me? I couldn't get it. It was like I was in the Twilight Zone.

I didn't know how to explain to her. I was certain we could have worked it out if she just spoke more softly, and slowly enough that I could follow. But it was obvious that she thought I was a troublemaker.

I was incapable of explaining that I had brain damage from the accident two days prior because I myself had no concept of what was wrong. And it never occurred to the office workers that my difficulties might be stemming from the accident.

I later found that it was important to smile and fake it at

times such as this—to nod and pretend that I understood, say "yes" often, and then try to work it out on my own later.

I gave up and left the office.

This was the first of many such situations in which people took offense at my manner as I struggled to navigate social situations, and got angry at me.

I drove home, and then rested through the evening, night, and next day, mostly staring at the wall, sitting in my Eames chair.

By Thursday I was feeling more normal, and taught my class downtown at DePaul. Because I couldn't read more than a line or two, I lectured extemporaneously from memory—while sitting at the desk in front of the class. By the end of the lecture I was in the soup again, unable to stand or walk. One of my students drove me home.

Once back in my house, I tried to sleep, but I found that if I closed my eyes, or turned off the light, I got seasick from disorientation. In the end I fell asleep with my eyes open and the light on, staring at a spot on the wall.

By Friday I felt that I had lost control, and thought I had better go to the emergency room after all. But this was easier said than done. I had always been a natural multitasker: able to get my kids out the door and into the car, work on an AI problem in the back of my mind, consider the best route to our destination, make a mental note to call a friend, and so on, all running in parallel. Now I found that I could only do *one thing at a time*. If I had even the slightest thought about any other subject at all—for example, about where I was going, or what I was going to do there, or even simply *did I have my wallet?*—everything else just stopped dead: my body stopped moving, my balance systems began to fail, and my internal organization of keys, glasses, doors, coats, and shoulder bags disappeared into the ether.

DO YOU KNOW YOUR NAME?

On my way to the emergency room I drove along a thoroughfare I had traveled daily for eighteen years. But nothing was
familiar to me, and none of the landmarks in the visual scene
carried any meaning. I was not delusional. I could have described, for example, the middle school that my daughter attended, and identified it by name. But the description would
have been purely intellectual in nature. There was nothing
about my visual apprehension of the actual school building
that would lead me to believe I had ever seen it before. There
would be no visceral sense it inspired, no history, and I could
not use it in the visual-spatial scene for navigation because it
had no "place information" attached to it. In a Capgras-like
twist (a delusion in which family members seem to have been
supplanted by look-alikes), it was as though all the buildings

had been replaced by others that looked the same, but were part of a foreign landscape that was not my home.

With difficulty I managed to get myself admitted to the emergency room, but I have only patchy memories from the seven hours I spent at the hospital. The intake nurses asked me questions, but I couldn't make sense of them. Later, in a scene reminiscent of a late-night horror movie I was rolled around in a wheelchair, overcome with nausea from the motion, and the spinning of the visual scene in front of my eyes, as I went through batteries of tests. The orderly who was pushing me kept banging my foot into things; it hurt, but I couldn't figure out how to ask him not to do that anymore. I had specifically rehearsed three things that I wanted to make sure the doctor knew when I finally got to talk to him, but I couldn't retrieve even one of them sufficiently to be able to form the necessary words.

The doctor asked me, "Do you know what your name is?" I could see, in my mind's eye, the words "Dr. Clark Elliott" in black type against a white rectangular background, mixed case, in Times New Roman font. However, as soon as I started to speak the answer, the words disappeared. But the vocalization had only just started. Without the words before my eyes, my motor system failed, and I could not speak them. At this point I also found myself unable even to decide whether the answer was "yes" I *knew* what my name was—after all I could see it in front of my eyes—or "no" I was unable to perform what is known as the *speech act* of saying my name in response to the question.

In the end I just sputtered.

I was so frustrated that my eyes filled with tears. I felt that the doctor assumed I was just an idiot. I felt like I was faking it somehow, in a perverse scheme to emphasize my troubles. But I was not an idiot. I knew exactly what was going on (sort of, in one way). I just couldn't communicate it. I wanted to have the doctor understand my symptoms, and wanted to be an active participant in treatment, but was completely shut out of the process.

Much later, when they were ready to discharge me, the doctor simply said, "Everything looks fine." I asked him, "What's the problem? I don't feel right." He said, "You have a concussion, and it's a bad one." I remember seeing the words "severe concussion" written on a form.

The doctor told me I could go home, then left. They gave me some papers, which turned out to be instructions telling me to have someone wake me up several times at night, but I didn't read them until months later. I didn't know what they were, I was living by myself, and besides, by this time I had found that I couldn't read. They gave me some pills, but I didn't know what to do with them. (I discovered the bottle of Vicodin in a drawer, unopened, a year later.)

It would have been extremely helpful to have some explanation given, carefully, of what a concussion was. That is, something such as, "You have permanent brain damage and it is going to take some time for your brain to rewire itself to work around the trouble so that you can start to function more normally. In the meantime—for months—you might expect to have a lot of trouble getting through the day." But no such explanation was given, and I was simply given my clothes and released. It took me several hours to make the one-mile drive home.

By the next morning my arm was quite sore. By Sunday it was swollen to twice its size. The hospital staff had forgotten to take the catheter out of my arm before releasing me. It would have been easy for me just to take the tape off and pull the catheter needle out, which any reasonable person would have done. But I couldn't make sense of it: my arm hurt . . . it was swollen . . . I had been in the hospital. . . . For some reason there was tape and a plastic connector, with a big needle sticking in my arm. I couldn't figure out how to get the tape off. The best I could manage was to drive back to the hospital emergency room one-handed and bang on the glass door with my good arm.

It was after midnight, so the overnight guard sent me in to the nurses' desk. The nurse there laughed when she saw my arm, and others of the night staff, standing around the nurses' station, looked over our way, and started laughing too, at my expense. I was the big joke that night—too goofy to realize I had a needle sticking in my arm. I felt both helpless and ashamed to be such a dope with my swollen arm. My sense of isolation was growing.

WORD MAPS GONE AWRY

By this time, because the experiences were so odd—and, in a macabre way, fascinating to me as an AI scientist—I had taken to capturing the most salient details on scraps of paper around the house, and in short text files on my computer, stuffed into random directories. It was ironic that I could not read, but as long as I did not go back over my work, or think about what I was saying, I could write after a fashion, consistent with my odd, fractured brain state. Trying to read would leave me in pain, and wear me out within a few minutes. By contrast, if I just let my fingers produce the sentences directly from the images in my head, I could write for twenty minutes or more at a time. The key was to *not see the words*.

This turned out to be a general theme in my life as a concussive: my creativity was actually enhanced—both by my need to invent novel solutions to tricky problems that now continually arose in everyday life, and also, in a perverse way, by damage to the perceptual filters that most of us use to block out much of the detail in the world around us. For someone like me whose filters weren't working, those observed details could sometimes lead to creative ways of seeing solutions that others might miss.*

To outsiders it looked, on the surface, as though my life were continuing as it had prior to the crash. Because of my recent divorce, I had purchased a burned-out house in a neighborhood close to where my children lived, and, making use of my experience as a former boat builder and carpenter, I was rebuilding it. After the crash, I made my teaching at the university a critical priority, second only to being a father. My young children were with me a little less than half of the time, and the rest of the time I lived alone. As I was able, I continued to manage the subcontractors who were often in and out of my house.

My personality was such that I tended to keep quiet about my struggles and see if I could work them out on my own. My mother often joked that the first words out of my mouth as a toddler were, "Do it myself! Do it myself!"

But I couldn't hide everything.

One of the problems that started to arise, and that ultimately I had to be quite vigilant about, was that while writing I would use inappropriate words in odd places. At times this was so

---

*It turns out that there is a strong link between people who dispositionally exhibit this failure to filter out extraneous information (in a syndrome known as *cognitive disinhibition*) and highly creative thought. See, e.g., Shelley Carson, "The Unleashed Mind: Why Creative People Are Eccentric," *Scientific American Mind*, April 14, 2011, http://www .scientificamerican.com/article.cfm?id=the-unleashed-mind. See also references for Schizotypal Personality [disorder].

peculiar that I feared appearing mentally ill to others in my professional life. My notes and e-mail messages from the time show that I frequently had begun incorrectly substituting words in my writing that *sounded* similar, or, sometimes, that were *conceptually* similar. For example: over-serving/(instead of) observing, way/weigh, right/write, imagine/manage, say/said, feeling/meaning, phone perception/phone reception. Sometimes I would get phrases wrong, such as "yet to be reader"/"yet to be written," and "wrapped tightly under practice"/"wrapped tightly under plastic."

I believe that many of these errors had to do with my inability to do two things at once, and would happen when my mind strayed momentarily to an ancillary thought. In one example, while composing an e-mail response, I noted that I was thinking of a "file" where text about a tenure meeting was stored. The "f" from file caused "meeting" to become "feeting," which was subconsciously corrected to "feeling," thus producing the phrase "tenure feeling" in place of "tenure meeting."

I had different difficulties with spoken English.

According to my brother's observations, which he made during a rare visit a year after the crash, I would "talk . . . like . . . this . . . ," with my eyes staring out of focus, and my head tracing slow arcs through the space around me, as though I were trying to *will* the words to come to visual consciousness, or trying to locate them in the space around me, searching for them in slow motion.

WHY ARE YOU HERE?

Several weeks after the crash I was feeling so debilitated and confused that I again called the family doctor, and again was told to go to the emergency room.

I was understandably reluctant to return to the hospital, but I was getting desperate. I couldn't make sense of what was happening to me. By this time a whole potpourri of strange things had been occurring. I would get stuck in a chair, unable to get up for an hour at a time. I could go up stairways, but I could not go down them. I couldn't understand jokes that people told. I couldn't follow announcers on the radio. I often had to sleep with my eyes open. I had serious balance problems. Shopping was almost impossible. I couldn't take the train, or manage an elevator. I couldn't listen to anyone on the phone for more than a minute or two before nausea began to set in.

The emergency room was busy. After waiting forty minutes, I was taken inside and told to take my clothes off, put on a gown, and lie down on a bed. This took me a long time. The geometry of my clothing was difficult for me to "see," and consequently my hands were moving in slow motion, and awkwardly.

A harried emergency room nurse came in to talk to me.

"Why did you come here?" she asked.

"I don't know why I came," I said honestly. "I don't know what's wrong."

She looked at me suspiciously. "How can we help you, if you won't tell me why you are here?"

She was right, but I didn't know what to do. So I didn't say anything.

"Dr. Elliott, have you been taking drugs? Did you take something? Have you been drinking?"

I shook my head, but didn't say anything.

She left, and sometime later, a doctor came in. Presumably he had looked me up, and seen that I had been diagnosed recently with a concussion. He had a clipboard with him.

"Are you in pain?" he asked.

"Yes," I said. "A lot of pain." This was true. Whenever I had had to think about anything the pain in my head and in the neck muscles under my skull was intense. "Strange things have been happening to me."

"Do you have nausea?" he asked.

"Yes," I said. "If I try to read, or think about much of anything at all, I have to work hard to keep from throwing up."

"Okay," he said, and wrote something on the clipboard without any explanation. Then he left. I lay on the bed and stared at the cloth curtain that separated me from the next bed.

The nurse returned after a while. I sat up and she put a small paper cup with some pills in it in my hand. She said something to me, but she was talking very fast because they were busy, and I couldn't process what she said. I didn't understand what to do with the pills, so I just lay back on the bed, holding them in my hand, working hard trying to understand the situation. I could see that the pills were two different shapes, and I didn't know what that meant. I didn't know what was going on, what I was supposed to do, or what was going to happen.

After forty-five minutes the nurse came back. She was upset that I still had the pills in my hand. I believe the idea was that I was to have taken the pills, and they would wait for them to take effect and see how I was doing.

"Oh, good grief," she said. "What are you doing? Why didn't you take the pills? We've got a lot of really sick people here." My head hurt at the sound of her harsh words.

So I swallowed the pills (one for nausea, and one for the head pain?). In retrospect, I guess the nurse just saw me as a malingerer who wouldn't follow instructions and was taking up a bed needed for someone with a broken leg. I put my clothes back on, accepted some papers, and left.

It took me half an hour to figure out how to get back to the garage and find my car. (This is a two-minute trip ordinarily—the emergency room is next to the garage.) I couldn't make sense of the hospital corridors; it was hard for me to get up the stairs because I couldn't "see" them; I didn't understand the geometry of the parking garage; I had to hold on to the walls for balance. When I finally found the Mazda, I was exhausted. So I sat in the driver's seat with the door open, just resting, waiting until it was safe for me to drive.

But I had no luck. After twenty minutes the security guard came and told me he had seen me prowling around the garage, and if I didn't leave immediately he was going to have me arrested.

And even though I had done nothing wrong, in my weakened condition I really did fear that this might happen: I looked disheveled, I was acting as if I was perhaps on drugs, I was sitting in a car with a smashed-in rear end, and it would be hard for me to explain my circumstances—not exactly a person to inspire confidence as the cream of society. With the unfamiliar shapes, the stress, and the noise, jail would be more than I could manage.

Alarmed, I mustered the energy to drive out of the parking garage, and stopped down the street, where I rested and contemplated my strange condition. I finally got home three hours later.

I felt much worse than when I had gone to the hospital in the first place, and also now knew definitively that the emergency room was not an option that was going to help. I was on my own on this one.

Not surprisingly, I vowed never to return to the hospital. And I never did.

APPLE, SCARF, TREE

Despite my difficulties with planning, I did manage, finally, during this period to make contact with a local neurology group. At the prompting of the family doctor, I had tried to see an established neurologist, but the soonest one could see me was in two months. I was reluctant to wait this long, fearing that I was possibly sustaining further damage to my brain— my symptoms were so strange, and not getting better. The office could "squeeze me in," they said, in three weeks with a neurologist who had just joined their practice.

I spent a day carefully writing out notes on exactly what I had been experiencing, which I now know to be classic symptoms of concussion, but which, apparently, were not of interest to most physicians at the time. I used up another morning getting the notes into a stamped and addressed envelope to be picked up by the postman, to be read in advance of my appointment.

On the day of my consultation I arrived well rested, and had done nothing the least bit taxing since the day before. I wanted to be at my best.

"Good morning, Dr. Elliott," said the middle-aged neurologist. "I understand you are concerned about a concussion? Tell me, were you in an automobile accident? Is there a lawsuit? Were you wearing your seat belt?"

These were standard questions asked of me by virtually every physician I saw. We can suppose there are often, on the one hand, annoying troubles from lawyers that make extra work for physicians, and, on the other hand, lucrative expert witness fees when there are lawsuits. It also seems to be the case, to me, that there is *always* an assumption that if there is an automobile accident, there will be lawsuit money, and thus everyone is immediately suspicious that you are faking it.

I told him there was no lawsuit.

He then gave me a variation of a thirty-question test called the *Folstein Mini–Mental State Examination.*

"What is today's date?" he began. "Can you tell me what season it is?"

I did fine at the beginning of the test.

"Okay. Good. Now remember these three objects: an *apple*, a *scarf*, and a *tree.* Can you repeat them back to me?"

"Sure. Apple, um . . . scarf, and, uh, um . . . tree."

He then had me count backward by sevens from one hundred. This was quite stressful because of the sequencing and the visualization, which, as we will see, were very challenging for me. I had only been with the doctor for a few minutes but I was starting to feel strange and disoriented again, in the way that was becoming quite familiar.

"One hundred, ninety-three, . . . eighty-six, . . . , . . . seventy-nine, . . . , . . . , . . . seventy-two," I said, getting slower and slower as I progressed. I could feel my tongue getting heavy, and I began to lose my balance as I sat in the chair.

"Okay, fine," said the doctor. "Now tell me the three objects again."

"Um, uh, apple," I said.

"Go on!" he said in a commanding voice.

"Ah . . . ah . . . ," I said. I could see the scarf in my mind's eye, but as soon as I tried to say the word, the image went blank, and I couldn't speak. My eyes were staring. I was getting increasingly nauseated. "Scarf," I finally managed.

"GO ON!" he said in an even louder voice.

But I couldn't manage it.

He now started to verbally abuse me. "Say the word!" he shouted. "TELL ME THE THIRD WORD! THREE items, not TWO!"

It was as though I could either "see" the word in my mind's eye, or say it, but not both. I was having trouble understanding even the concept of there being *three* items. His shouting felt like I was being beaten in the head. I recalled the image of a tree, but then the word "Tree" began to blend together with the word "Three," which was similar. I was drowning in sensory and cognitive input.

"Tree," I finally managed.

He made notations in my file. Then he gave me a simple drawing exercise to complete.

"Do you see," I said, "that I am now having trouble with

motor coordination, with controlling my hands?" I was doing my best, but by now drawing very slowly.

He didn't say anything, but instead waited for me to complete the drawing. He wasn't interested in what I had to say.

He then gave me a physical exam that specifically included reflex testing, banging me below my knees and near my elbows.

At the end of the exam, which had lasted about fifteen minutes, he said, "You are fine. I don't see any real problem here. I think if you rest for a few days, you'll be okay."

But I felt far from fine. And I had done nothing *but* rest for weeks. The simple mental exercises he had given me were specifically very difficult, and had left my cognitive state seriously depleted. I was moving in slow motion. I was becoming unable to filter sensory information.

On leaving the office I avoided the elevator because I did not want to have to deal with the disorientation I knew would result. But then I got stuck at the top of the stairwell. I couldn't "see" the stairs. I gave up and sat down on the top step, unable to proceed. It took me forty-five minutes to get down the single flight of stairs, moving from step to step, holding on to the wall, and another hour to manage the short drive home.

I was no closer to understanding what was happening to me. The doctor had said I was fine, but everything was still so difficult for me.

Given what I know now from my own experience, and from talking with other concussives, there was critical information missing from that exam. First, in a theme that would come up again in the future, had the cognitive exams been given to me a second time I would not have been able to complete them, because a signature of my concussion was the rapid cognitive deterioration that took place under certain kinds of cognitive stress. That is, I would present as almost normal for a few minutes, but then would fall off a "cliff," so to speak, under the cumulative mental load. Yet, in my experience, standard medical procedure never calls for repeating these types of exams. Second, in another theme that would come up in my interactions with medical professionals, there was no baseline set for a patient's raw cognitive intelligence or education—which can be crucial information in determining what deficits have occurred. Third, the onset of balance difficulties and the deterioration of motor skills during the exam should have been a dead giveaway.

In short, at the time, the standard neurologists' response to concussion was to give me an exam designed for dementia, and, my having passed that, and a simple set of reflex tests, send me home.

A week later, the neurologist sent a letter to the family doctor suggesting that I get a little more rest before teaching my classes. He completely missed both the nature of, and the extent of, my impairment.

I was so enraged by the letter's cavalier treatment of my difficulties, and also by the fact that the doctor appeared not to have even bothered to read through the careful list of symptoms I had sent him—and which, in my condition, had taken me so much effort to prepare—that I composed a draft of a detailed response letter complaining about his commentary. As a professor, I was disappointed that he would be so unscientific—his conclusions didn't match the facts. But I never sent it. I couldn't manage the details of getting the letter into an envelope, stamped, addressed, and into a mailbox.

So my immediate options had run out. It happened to be the case that as a cognitive scientist, I found my symptoms interesting, and it also happened to be in my nature that I just seldom gave up when I was pursuing the solution to some hard problem, consistent with my work at the university. So I kept at it for almost a decade, without the slightest encouragement that I'd ever get better. In fact, I heard repeatedly from various branches of the medical profession that after a certain point I would *not* get better, that *no one ever did.*

But we have to ask, how many other concussives have simply given up at this point? Virtually every "expert" I had seen had shown little interest in my condition, and even less understanding. I had been treated with suspicions that I was a malingerer, a troublemaker, and perhaps even a scam artist. I had no idea what had happened to me, and didn't even, really, understand that there was anything seriously wrong with me. I thank my stars that at least I was not diagnosed as a mental case and treated with psychotropic drugs.

Given my experiences, I am certain that there are thousands of people in the United States alone still needlessly going through exactly the same misadventures that I did. They'll have no understanding of what has happened to them. They might find that cognitive treatments are not covered by medical insurance, or recognized by the armed forces, or understood by their physicians. They'll run into hostility and the suspicion that they are faking it, or that they have mental problems. They may end up paying for treatments that don't address the root of the problem, and listening to well-meaning professionals' unfortunate conclusions, then go home to live with their condition for the rest of their lives because they have nowhere else to turn.

PART TWO
THE COMPONENTS
OF COGNITION

In this section of the book, we will focus on the important *cognitive themes* that defined my concussion experience over the next eight years. How was I able to manage such severe symptoms, and yet still keep my job? What was the relationship between my visual system problems and my balance difficulties? Why was it that one day I couldn't walk across a parking lot, but the next I could run a marathon? Why couldn't I read anymore?

BACKGROUND

Despite the obvious challenges, I was in many ways blessed by the *structure* of my life, both at work and at home.

Very important to this story is my employer, DePaul University—our nation's largest Catholic university—which afforded me critical flexibility in my work schedule, and thus allowed me to continue working as a professor. DePaul is quietly one of the little-known jewels in the academic world. Faculty positions were—and are—highly sought after by those (like me) who believed in a strong commitment to both teaching and service in such an eclectic environment—in addition to their pure research—because this meant that there were many ways for us to make a contribution to the university. This emphasis on a broader kind of service to the academic community allowed me further flexibility in how I could approach my job. I was surrounded by peers who were high-quality researchers, but also, in this unique academic environment, universally good teachers as well. This ubiquitous "teaching personality" generally made them curious about, and sensitive to, the idiosyncrasies of others—including me. My students, too, were both thoughtful and helpful in working around my impairments. The service-oriented Vincentian ethics of the school provided a trickle-down grounding that fostered the well-being of its faculty, staff, and students, and thus wrapped me in a very supportive environment.* And, too, I was part of the hugely vibrant College of Computing and Digital Media, which has sported, for many years, one of the largest graduate programs in computer science in the world, giving me a great deal of flexibility in the courses I could teach. I was *very* lucky to be at DePaul.

My faculty peers were understanding. The dean of my school was compassionate, and strategic about making the best use of my diminished skills. I scaled back my promising international research career in computing emotions and instead focused on collecting and developing ideas for much later publication. I emphasized service to the college and my teaching.

At the time of the crash I was, after two decades, away from the stress of a long-failing marriage. I had my own place to live. Except for some initial difficulties in getting to see my older children, life was on the upswing. It was, overall, a time of great promise. My natural exuberance for life was still intact. I was surprised to find that, even after only a few hours of something like sleep, I woke up almost every morning thinking, *Hmm—how about that, another good day!*

---

*This commitment to service really is pervasive, and starts at the top: the Reverend Dennis H. Holtschneider, C.M., Ed.D., president of DePaul, for example, donates his entire $800,000-plus salary to the Vincentian order, of which he is a member.

I only gradually began to realize—after a fashion—that my life was significantly changed and that this was not just some temporary state, like having the flu. After all, as long as I didn't *think*, I looked and felt pretty much normal. And when I did have to think, I became so engrossed in solving the immediate resulting problems that I didn't have room for making a global assessment of my circumstances. It was just one foot after another, every hour, every day.

It's true that I was daily encountering strange and difficult problems to solve. But solving hard, novel problems—mostly on my own—was for me a way of life, both personally and professionally. It was, in many ways, just business as usual. The work was similar; the problems were different.

A month before the crash I had moved into a small, burned-out house with only limited power and plumbing, which I was intent on rebuilding. I lived there alone, except when my older children were visiting. After sustaining the concussion I continued to work at the construction with various subcontractors as I was able, with no choice but to finish much of the job myself over the course of several years.

I had many big hearts around me during that difficult time. I formed what are now ongoing thirteen-year bonds with my second wife, Qianwei—a Chinese computer scientist—and my deeply thoughtful stepdaughter Lucy, with each of whom I remain close, despite de facto separation starting in 2006. Qianwei's parents lived with us for a year, during which time they became grandparents to our enchanting daughter Erin (my youngest), who has lived with me her entire life—including mostly having me as a single parent from the time she was two years old. Nell, the oldest of my three children from my first marriage (the *rocket girl*, who has been unfailingly supportive of me), has been with me most of her life—and exclusively so from early high school through the completion of her master's degree at Brown University in *combinatorial optimization*. Peter, my second, lives close by, and has visited with me off and on. Lucy, my third by age, was always with me, even when her mom was frequently out of the country on long business trips. Paul, my fourth (who was crucial in getting me through my most difficult challenges with his little sister, and who often just *helped* with whatever I needed at the time), spent almost half his time at my house. So, during this entire period I was often the single parent for a houseful of bright and thoughtful children.

My good friend Jake, who also figures prominently in this narrative, lived nearby in Chicago until he moved to take a job in San Diego in 2002, where he continued to support me remotely.

Although none of the treatments I pursued ever helped with any of the actual root causes of my brain problems during this eight-year period, I kept hacking away at it, leaving no stone unturned, so to speak, in looking for such help. In addition to my visits to the emergency room, and to the first neurologist, I later visited a nationally known rehabilitation center, a balance clinic, a neurotherapy clinic, a homeopath, various M.D.s, and had every diagnostic psychological test available at the time. I saw two prestigious neurologists and a psychiatrist. All of these practitioners and institutions were serious about their work. Some of my visits were informational—which in itself was helpful to me—but beyond that, no one had anything to offer a TBI victim beyond compassion and the suggestion that I learn to live with my permanent symptoms.

Additionally, I had some success with various treatments

from an electrostimulation therapist, an orthopedic physical therapist who specialized in brain injuries, a standard chiropractor, an Atlas-specialty chiropractor, an herbalist, an acupuncturist, and a sports-medicine specialist. Each helped me to somewhat manage my symptoms, and to persevere. I studied Tai Chi for many years, with a gifted and deeply spiritual teacher who had a profound effect on my ability to experience joy in my much-altered life, and to manage the physical pain. Lastly, I had several years of deep massage with a superb Chicago therapist. His treatment was a godsend for the pain, and always helped, temporarily, to restore some cognitive function.

But, again, none of these avenues of treatment, no matter how effective at briefly addressing my *symptoms*, helped with the brain injury itself.

Besides simple survival, my main task during the years after sustaining my concussion was to figure out the *principles of my impairment* so that I could conserve my resources and make it through the week. Which activities were the most taxing, and why? What were the rules behind the complex interplay of sensory input, brain-body states, and human cognition? Gradually, themes began to emerge—captured here in the ten broad categories that make up this section of the book.

We will consider each of these topics as essential in understanding the cognitive breakdowns occurring in a damaged brain, but should also see them as a unique set of windows onto the fascinating workings of the *healthy* human brain as well. We'll look at many facets of what makes us human at some of the lowest levels of our cognitive machinery. Then, at the close of this part of the book, we'll meet *the Ghost*, who ushered in the period of my miraculous recovery almost a decade after the crash.

THE HUMAN MACHINE IS BROKEN

THE THREE LEVELS OF COGNITIVE BATTERIES. Under certain circumstances, for varying but generally short periods of time, I would appear to act—and respond to challenges—normally. Then, under what would appear to outsiders as identical circumstances, I became reluctant and difficult instead. Others in my personal and professional life began to see me as sometimes unaccountably unreliable, or even obstructionist. Frustrated with my own fluctuations, I began to see myself that way as well.

It was hard to explain why it was possible for me to grade one exam in ten minutes, but it took all day to grade five of them; or why one minute I could converse freely about a complex unification algorithm used in AI programs, but ten minutes later couldn't understand what "next Tuesday at 4:15" meant.

Gradually I began to see a pattern. As long as I did not have to *think* and could avoid certain kinds of tasks, and if there were no demands on my balance system, I was more or less functional. The more I used my brain over the course of minutes or hours, the less functional I became. And the rate of my deterioration was highly dependent on the *kind* of brain activity I was performing: Trying to process two streams of simultaneous input (such as talking on the phone while jotting down notes on the conversation), making decisions, or sorting out the visual landscape when shopping, would leave me incapacitated within a few minutes. Performing simpler activities, such as driving, washing dishes, and socializing that did not involve attending to significant conversation, did not cause deterioration. Over time, I learned to make reasonable predictions about my cognitive and sensory breakdowns based on the kinds of thinking activities I had to perform, and on the current state of my brain resources.

Equally important were the varying rates at which I could *recover* from my distress.

Understanding the relationship between these two—the ways that breakdowns occurred, and the different speeds with which I recovered from them—is critical to understanding many of the otherwise puzzling episodes that I so often experienced. Nor was my experience unique: other concussives I spoke to over the years had exactly the same perplexing difficulty. Over time I found myself using a *cognitive battery* analogy to capture the structure of this recurring breakdown and recovery phenomenon:

Imagine that a concussive has three sets of batteries that power her brain. *Set A*—the working set—is immediately available, and also recharges rapidly within a few hours. *Set*

B—the first level of backup batteries—can be accessed if Set A is exhausted, but takes longer to recharge, possibly up to several days. *Set C*—the deepest level of backup batteries—can be used as a last resort at times of extreme demand when Set B is exhausted. But caution must be exercised—Set C charges very slowly, over the course of up to two weeks.

Now here is the problem—it is not possible for our concussive to charge Set B very well until Set C is fully charged, and similarly it is not possible to charge Set A very well until Set B is fully charged. So, once Set C has been drained, it is going to be a long time until our concussive's brain returns to (relatively) "normal" operation.

As long as our concussive can get by using her Set A batteries to power her brain, life will be relatively normal. But this means that her brain can only be used for short periods, and not in ways that are very demanding. These short shallow-demand periods must also be interspersed with regular brain rest—and often, in particular, *visual system* rest. The concussive needs periods of doing nothing, without thinking, or dreaming, or taking action.

But, life intrudes. Some tasks require that our concussive stay focused for longer periods, or require more intense use of her brain than can be powered by the Set A batteries. Going shopping, for example, requires that she perform extensive pattern matching and decision making. Caring for children requires that she always be prepared to respond, even when it is not convenient. At these times the Set A batteries are rapidly used up, and the concussive has to draw on the Set B batteries to power her cognition. Even so, as long as there is a period of several days during which she can recover, life will return to "normal."

The real problems begin when the Set B batteries are used up, and there is not sufficient time for them to be recharged. Something comes up—say that after returning from an exhausting shopping trip one of the children discovers that he has left his expensive eyeglasses in one of the stores—our concussive has to respond, and as a last resort, she dips into her emergency energy source: the Set C batteries. These work fine, but only for a very short period of time. Using them, our concussive appears normal, and seems to act normally, in responding to the demanding circumstances. But when the Set C batteries are used up, there is nothing else for our concussive to draw on. Her life will not return to "normal" without a week or two of rejuvenating cognitive rest while the Set C batteries recharge.

In my case, this odd, terraced way that my cognitive batteries drained, and recharged, was both a godsend and a curse. On the one hand, it was a blessing because it allowed me, for example, to drive safely, knowing that if some driving situation occurred, requiring that I respond to a series of challenges, I would be able to draw on reserves to react appropriately; it allowed me to keep my job by being mentally present at important meetings that were cognitively challenging; it allowed me to reasonably get through conversations in important social situations. Most important, it allowed me to be an effective parent: if my children needed me, I could step in and take over in a responsible way.

On the other hand, it was a curse because outsiders might look at me doing fine on some task and expect that I would always be able to perform it, and others like it, not realizing the extreme toll it was taking.

Lastly, independent of what I've described as the three

levels of cognitive batteries, there was another, different, effect I could call on. This "extreme emergency" mode could be called up in an instant, to deal with dangerous situations typically associated with rushes of adrenaline, and could usually support "normal" body and cognitive functioning for a very short time—as long as the Set C batteries still had *some* reserve. However, it was exceedingly draining, always took a heavy toll, and required a significant recovery period.

While "deep C battery" mode and "extreme emergency" mode are a godsend to the concussive, acting as emergency buffers, they are not to be taken lightly: from the perspective of the residual emotional/physical trauma they engender, drawing on those deep emergency batteries starts out roughly equivalent to shouting at a child that a big wave is coming, or jamming on the car brakes, and quickly moves up to something more like reaching into a fire to retrieve an important document, or jumping off a roof to avoid danger.

How long did it take for the various battery sets to deteriorate? This does not have a simple answer, because it depended on the tasks being executed at the time. Working up in a tree with a chain saw—which requires intense balance calculations, complex visual pattern matching on both the moving background of the gently rocking tree and the fluttering leaves, and extreme vigilance so an arm or leg does not get cut off, will almost immediately work through Sets A and B, and soon start to carve deeply into the resources of Set C. Twenty minutes in a tree with a chain saw is guaranteed to require a week of rest to get fully back to relative equilibrium. By contrast, being the single parent of a continually chattering three-year-old will slowly exhaust the battery supply over the course of several weeks, because there is just never any chance for the brain to rest and recover.

A few years after the crash a neurologist told me, "You won't get any better—after two years, no one ever does. But you'll get better at figuring out ways to live with your brain damage." He was right about the last part. I grew quite crafty about avoiding cognitive and sensory activities that drained my batteries. In this way I sometimes appeared socially odd ("Goddammit, Elliott, why isn't your voicemail turned on!"), but was otherwise able to present a reasonably normal façade to the outer world.

I suspect that many concussives use similar techniques in their lives. So, while their brains may not have recovered, with time they have nonetheless become more adept at compensating for their impairments by avoiding debilitating activities. And, yes, this avoidance behavior will often make them seem irritable, or touchy, or just plain *weird*.

GETTING STUCK AND THE MAGIC OF INITIATION. One great thing that our bodies do for us, and which we never think about, is to *initiate action*. An important element of this is the concept of our spatial sense—our knowledge of who we are within the space around us.* The way this works is: we want to look at an item, or pick it up, or walk over to where it is, and the next thing we know we are turning our head to look at it, or reaching for it, or moving our legs to walk to it. But, as we have seen from my adventure getting home from work that winter night, there is a moment we never think about when

---

*A cognitive sense, thought to be located in the superior parietal lobe.

"magic" happens, when thought is translated into action, and we make the almost instantaneous transition from being still to being in motion.

Concussives often lose the ability to make that transition.

It is easy to imagine yourself in such circumstances: You are completely comfortable. You are not physically tired. You really, actually, want to rise up out of your chair, and you might even say the words, "Okay, let's go now." But as you stare off into space wondering why this is happening . . . nothing moves. It is an odd sensation. It is not at all like being numb—you can feel every part of your body, the same as always. It is not scary, the way you would feel if you were paralyzed. Instead it is like being so globally lazy that you just can't get yourself to *feel* like moving. It's like watching yourself sitting there doing nothing from the outside in.

There is a haziness about it too, as though you can't quite "get" what it would mean to actually move. You can't *see* it. In some strange and subtle way it's as though moving, and the comprehension of moving, belongs to an alternate, unknowable universe.

For someone who studies the implementation of artificial intelligence, this can spark a marvelous moment of insight: if you can't "see" where you are going, or the thing you want to reach for—see your target's place, and *your* place, within the visual/spatial representation of the world around us that we all keep in our heads—then your muscles simply will not move. Your low-level motor-control system doesn't respond to words; it responds to *spatial images*. It is all very elemental, complex, useful, pragmatic . . . and it all happens for us without thought, in the blink of an eye.

Being unable to move can be embarrassing, and socially difficult. I learned to plan ahead. Sometimes I'd just avoid walking down stairs (which were particularly problematic), attending meetings, and making decisions, any of which might get me stuck. Other times, I'd tell a trusted colleague or student of mine that "I'm going to likely have a little trouble after [the meeting/class]," and ask him or her, "Would you be kind enough to pull me up out of my chair and push me out of the room when we are done?" Fortunately, once I *got* moving I was usually okay.

I learned to be humble enough to simply ask strangers, "I'm working around a brain injury—could you possibly give me a little push so I can get going down the Jetway here?"*

Sometimes I only needed someone to *command me* to initiate the action. In the strangest of my workarounds I could literally tell someone exactly what to tell *me* to do. I could then follow their commands to initiate actions that I couldn't manage on my own. In the most baroque of these scenarios, I would call my friend Jake on the phone to have him get me unstuck.

Me: "Hi, Jake. Sorry. I've been here for twenty minutes. I need you to tell me to get up out my chair and walk into the kitchen."

Jake (in an authoritative voice): "Okay, Clark—GET UP OUT OF YOUR CHAIR NOW AND WALK ACROSS THE ROOM."

Me: "Thanks. I'm up now."

Jake: "No problem. Bye."

---

*For those concussives reading this, looking for tips, I'll note: it was harder to ask women, who apparently have to be more cautious about this kind of thing (though once they've committed they are more helpful); it was easier to ask a stranger for a push than a tug because the former seems to feel less personal.

Getting stuck, unable to move at all, is an important symptom of concussion. Many different problems, such as those of pattern matching, cognitive slow motion, decision making, and sensory overload, lead to this elemental breakdown in motor control.

THE MYSTERY OF CHOICE. Another troubling consequence of concussion may be the loss of the ability to make *decisions*. This has nothing to do with the ability to assess what a correct decision would be. Concussives have not become stupid or irrational. Rather it is the troubling loss of the *innate ability* to pull the trigger on a decision once the data has been collected and an analysis has been made.

Even within the general population, the facility with which people make decisions falls on a spectrum, and a concussive's loss of decision-making ability is best understood in context. We all know intelligent and organized people with good assessment skills who still, in the end—even after careful research— have trouble actually *deciding* what to do, whether it's buying a car or ordering dinner from a menu. We also know people who have little interest in researching facts prior to making a decision, and yet they have no trouble deciding on a path. Thus we can see that the native ability to decide—to pull the trigger at the crucial moment—has little general relationship to the amount of knowledge one has collected about the circumstances. Analysis and decision are two distinct processes.

If I hold up my hands and ask you to pick one, you'll have no trouble doing so. But here is the question: how did you choose? If you look closely, you'll realize that in all cases, independent of whether you do any preliminary work, at some point *magic happens*. A decision floats up from the ether inside your brain and action follows: pointing, speaking, reaching, and so on. Yet some concussives—during periods of brain fatigue—are incapable of such a seemingly simple task: you could offer them a thousand dollars to choose a hand—any hand—but they still might not be able to do so, because they can't *decide*.

This debilitating problem with decision making propagates throughout the whole system. The concussive's arm will not go up to "just pick one" without a clear visual/spatial instruction from the tired brain about where the arm is to reach. Phrases such as "the hand on the left" will not form without an image of *the hand on the left*, which is used to retrieve the words that make up the phrase. When a concussive looks inside her head for an answer, there is only an emptiness—like something perched, waiting along *with* her for the next step to occur. Those who have age-related trouble recalling nouns will have some sense of what this is like: you *know* you know the name of the movie actor to whom you wish to refer, but when you look inside to retrieve the name, nothing is there.

By January 2000—four months after the crash—I had grown increasingly brain-fatigued. My deep "cognitive batteries" were drained, and my life circumstances were such that I could not get the brain rest I needed for them to recover. I had not been able to manage shopping recently, so my food supplies were low. On one particular afternoon I was also hungry, with low blood sugar, which made matters worse.

Without thinking about it, I took an apple and some unsliced salami out of the refrigerator and placed them on my cutting board next to each other. I now had to decide: *Do I prepare the salami first, or the apple?*

Nothing came to mind. I was stuck, doing absolutely

nothing, waiting for a decision to arrive. From time to time thoughts would arise such as, *Just move your arm, you dope!* or *This is stupid. It makes absolutely no difference which one you prepare first.* But mostly I just stood there, hungry, staring at the food in front of me, waiting for the next step.

After fifteen minutes of staring at the food, getting nowhere, I gave up. Because of the intense effort I had made in trying to decide, I now had difficulty with motor control. Moving in slow motion, with contorted hands and shuffling feet, I returned the food to the refrigerator, and went away hungry. I had only made things worse: the need for a decision became ossified, centering around the two objects.

During the course of this particular incident (variations of which occurred over the months and years that followed), I returned to the kitchen ten times over the course of two days trying to get something to eat, like a rat repeatedly traversing a dead-end maze. Every visualization of a plan ended up in the same place: *then choose one.* Because I could not conceptualize what a decision was—could not *see it*—I had *no way to remove choice* from the alternate plans I formed.

After two days of forced fasting, and although I was loath to do it, I finally called Jake, and asked him to please instruct me to either eat the apple, or eat the salami. Jake's simple "Okay, go eat the salami first, then eat the apple"—just that one sentence, spoken over the phone, but which gave me a command to follow similar to that which allowed me to initiate physical motion— was enough to end the forty-eight hours of struggle.

KNOWING IS NOT CERTAINTY. People will talk about decisions as "gut-level feelings," and indeed decisions do seem to happen as a welling-up of action from the core of our being. Yet if most of us were to look closely at the actual process of making a decision, we would find that choices are usually represented with a visual/spatial metaphor, with two or more options laid out symbolically, such that particular features are shown in contrast along some spectrum. We might, for example, find ourselves choosing between the feel of "leftness versus rightness," "heaviness versus lightness," "peacefulness versus chaos," "intimacy versus expansiveness," or "wrongness (dark?) versus rightness (light?)," with colors, or shapes, or shadings, representing aspects of those concepts along a dimension.

The intellectual part of decision making, the "knowing" stage, is concerned with clarifying how the choices are represented, their various weights, and so on. Sometimes we might eliminate choices altogether by using logic.

But this is only the first part of the deciding process, and, surprisingly, is neither the most important, nor actually even necessary. (All people, in certain circumstances, can operate purely on intuition and skip the "knowing" stage altogether: "I don't know, just pick one and worry about it later!")

Much more critical is what follows. Once the choices have been captured in a symbolic, visceral, spatial way, *certainty* arises—or at least enough of it arises—and one of the choices is now marked within the 3D visual space as a goal. The body then responds by producing actions: a hand starts to reach for the apple, or the mind sees the words "Fine! I'll call her now . . ." and starts the vocalizing process to speak the words, and so on.

But this is the crucial step that is missing for the concussive with a fatigued brain: *certainty* never arises, the visual/spatial goal is never marked, and without a target the body cannot respond. No amount of inner dialogue from the "knowing" phase is of any help.

This is why the knowledge that either choice—eat the apple *or* the salami first—would be far better than no choice at all did not help me. It is also why the lack of a clear visual/spatial target left me physically stuck, unable to move, in exactly the same way I would get stuck at the top of stairs, or in trying to walk through a doorway: if I could not "see" the goal, my motor system could not respond.

Certainty also comes as a spectrum: you are completely certain that the sun came up this morning; you are reasonably certain that it was hot in Phoenix yesterday; you are somewhat certain that the Cleveland Indians will win the pennant this decade. There is a complex relationship between the degree of logically "knowing" something is likely to be true and the strength of certainty it generates—but the two are not always correctly linked, just as people sometimes use base rates correctly, and sometimes ignore them altogether.* Similarly, people will sometimes use the degree they *know* something to be true to create a like amount of certainty that it is; but sometimes they won't. Most people experience this as the difference between logic and intuition. In messy environments, especially when logical antecedents are incomplete—which is much of our world—informed intuition (enough certainty to allow us to act) is a critical part of our lives.

From an experiential standpoint, those who suffer from obsessive-compulsive disorder (OCD) often have similar problems: they might fully understand that they have already checked four times that the gas oven has been turned off; they might fully

---

*People will identify *correctly* a darting animal in their yard as a squirrel, not a platypus, because this is highly likely—they follow the base rates; they *incorrectly* fear mass murderers in schools when their children are vastly more likely to be harmed in a car accident—they don't follow the base rates.

understand that they are having an OCD attack and that return-ing once again to the house to check the oven is not going to help. But *knowing* does not help them, either. They too are missing that same elusive sense of certainty that drives the lower-level plan-ning system so closely tied to motor control. (And we should note that OCD is sometimes clearly linked to a previous TBI.)*

Elemental cognitive *certainty*—a concept easily understood but so elusive it defeats any attempt at formal algorithmic description—is a necessary component of many complex cog-nitive functions.

WHEN PIECES OF THE COGNITIVE MIND GO MISSING. Another difficult, insidious feature of concussion, and possibly the one that has most contributed to so many misdiagnoses and so much general misunderstanding of the condition, is that when cogni-tive capabilities go missing they are often so fully gone that the concussive does not miss them in the way a normal person would, or indeed sometimes even realize they've gone absent.

In my case, at the time when I was struggling with the apple, I was in the still-early phases of my post-concussion trauma. I didn't realize I had any kind of well-defined syndrome. I seemed unable to perform certain tasks, but outside of a vague uneasiness about the way things used to be, I had no real "sense" of the missing capabilities themselves.

Consider this analogy: You have a friend Joe, who for our purposes will represent a cognitive function that goes missing, such as decision making. If Joe moves to a monastery in

---

*From an anatomical perspective we might wonder if the *caudate nucleus* is missing crit-ical visual pattern-matching input that inhibits its ability to send suppression signals to the *cingulate gyrus* to tell it to stop sending anxiety triggers; an inappropriate balance between these two parts of the brain is suspected in OCD.

Thailand, you will know that you cannot call him to come over for a barbecue, and you might miss the interactions that you used to have with him. But you still know who he was, know how you *would* interact with him if he returned, and know exactly what is now missing from your life.

By contrast, for a concussive, when Joe moves to Thailand, it is as though he never lived at all. All relationships between Joe and anything else in the concussive's life have been removed, all memories of interaction with him are gone, and except for a vague, undifferentiated sadness for the way things used to be, there is no sense of missing *him*.

In this way—as I experienced during my unsuccessful ER visits—concussives are often unable to articulate what is wrong with them. *The cognitive machinery that is missing is also, exactly, the machinery necessary even to conceive of the machine itself.* In the case of the apple, the capability was easily described and easily understood: there are two objects, or paths of action, so pick one. Thus, intellectually, I *knew* what a decision was. But—and this is important to understand—I had no visceral *sense* of what a decision was. I had no feeling for what led up to the making of a decision except that magic used to happen, and now it no longer did.

NO LONGER HUMAN. This brings us, now, to one of the most troubling aspects of TBI, and one that we have to at least suspect is a significant contributor to the reported increase in the suicide rate among those of us with concussions: that we have, in many ways, already lost that which makes us *human*.* For a

---

*Isolating the causes of suicide is complex. Depression can lead to substance abuse problems. Substance abuse can lead to family problems. Concussion can lead to any of these; any can lead to an increase in suicide risk. However, we *can* say that "loss of self" is a critical risk factor, and that there is an increased risk of suicide after TBI.

concussive, no matter how long the list of *identified* cognitive deficits might become, there will still be hundreds of other small cognitive changes that are much less easy to define—though collectively they are perhaps even more important in the end.

This ubiquitous phenomenon is ultimately quite troubling for a concussive. For example, suppose you had lost the ability to naturally order your words as "the big blue box," instead of saying "the blue big box." Well, you would sort of know that something was wrong, and so would others, but exactly where is this syntactical preference capacity stored? A concussive is not privy to the internal workings of the brain, any more than anyone else is. It just *feels strange.* This kind of small breakdown happens all the time in so many ways—each contributing to the sense of alienation that many concussives share.

The net result is an overall feeling that we are no longer part of the human race: We look the same. We talk the same. People around us don't really notice too much difference. We haven't grown feebleminded, and the individual quirks that give us our essential personalities are all still in place. But inside, without really comprehending why, we are hugely changed. The person we have always known is strangely missing. This feeling is so pervasive among the concussives I've met over the years that it has become a standard private joke: *Welcome to life in exile. Welcome to life among the nonhumans.*

This feeling of being lost carries with it a sometimes terrible sadness—a longing to go home again, to taste again, just for a little while, the joys, and even sorrows, of being truly human just one more time. But, ultimately, it also carries with it the knowledge that the only way back is after first passing through the gates of death.

This is a dangerous combination. On the one hand, a concussive may feel that to a large extent he has already died. The step from life as a nonhuman to the ending of life altogether may not seem to matter very much. On the other hand, there is a longing to return home, to be human again. At some juncture, usually after the first two years have passed, most every concussive will finally approach the realization that in *this* life anyway, he is *never* going home again. When this happens, it is easy to imagine that finally shedding one's broken-down body—a body that can no longer support being human—might allow the spirit to return home on its own. Taken together we can see that in this way, for a concussive, pondering suicide might have nothing to do with a depressed and painful mental state, or being a cry for help, but rather a giving in, a simple final acknowledgment of what really, inside, has already happened. It is a walking *to*, instead of a walking *from*.

Another aspect of concussion that can be emotionally troubling is that the business of getting through the day just becomes so much work. As we've already seen in my own life, tasks that require any sort of visualization, or planning, or pattern matching, or balance, or decision making—in other words, more or less even the simplest things one might desire to do—become a struggle. Often a concussive will just want to put that burden down. Considering all the small battles fought just to get through a single day, life with concussion can feel like the labors of Sisyphus endlessly pushing his boulder up the hill.

On more than one occasion I wrote in my notes that I would have preferred to have lost two legs and one arm than to have suffered from concussion. I judged this to be a reasonable trade-off in my favor. At least I'd still be human.

BRAIN DAEMONS. In my academic field, artificial intelligence, there are two ways to simulate human intelligence: write computer programs using *human AI* techniques that attempt to model the actual processes of human thinking, or write programs using *alien AI* in which we write whatever sort of intelligent programs we feel like, as long as they get the job done, with no attempt to duplicate the way a human achieves the same goals. The former is typical of *cognitive science*, wherein we try to replicate the functional structures present in the brain. The latter captures the spirit of a device I'll use in this book, called *cognitive daemons*, wherein we simulate, and discuss, the effect of such processes on our lives, without regard to their real, underlying neural structure. That is, even without knowing how a human actually arranges to get more than one thing done at a time, using the simple computer science construct of a cognitive daemon allows us to accurately describe our feelings and behavior in a way that is easy to understand. In this way, even without proposing any neurological or anatomical models, we can nonetheless still claim that the design constraints on models of such systems, represented by my recorded experiences, are real.*

A *daemon*, for the purposes of our discussion, can be thought of as a "little guy that wakes up when needed to go perform some task, and reports back to you later with the results." Then he goes back to sleep (or dies off) until needed again. In the brain, what I refer to as daemons are thought processes that run independently, in the background (think, perhaps, of subconscious processing), and do their job over the course of

---

*That is, whatever we decide the real implementation of these processes is, any neurologically faithful daemons built from it will nonetheless still have to exhibit *all* the behavior we now independently describe.

seconds, minutes, days, or even weeks—working on some particular subproblem, and then interrupting conscious thought (or a different daemon) sometime in the future with their results. Sometimes daemons will spawn sub-daemons of their own.*

We cannot always control when these daemons get started; we can seldom control turning them off. A daemon tends to run its course—either solving the problem with which it has been tasked, or naturally and gradually giving up, as other problems take precedence. Daemons may be somewhat anxiety-driven, and slightly obsessive, as in "I just cannot remember that guy's name from California—the one who took us on his boat. What was that darn guy's name?"

Daemons run independently, but they can interfere with other, unrelated cognitions in at least two important ways: First, these background processes take up brain resources, leaving fewer resources for other processes, both conscious and subconscious. For example, if you are worried about your son's health, and in the back of your mind you are continually thinking about hypothetical diagnoses for his condition, you will appear preoccupied to others. You will perform less well on the other tasks in your life; you'll misplace your gloves and forget to feed your pet fish. This makes sense: there is only so much cognitive processing power to go around.

---

*In computer science, we have related constructs called *processes* that are used to implement the daemons. These constructs are similar to our daemon brain processing: they allow the computer to do many things at once, mostly in the background, of which the user is not aware. For example, a quick look at the list of computer tasks currently running on my laptop—which I am currently using only for the single, simple, "conscious" task of editing this book—shows that there are eighty-one other processes now running in the background: checking for network connectivity, updating my file index search function, listening for new USB connections, and so on.

Second, these background daemons appear to communicate with other parts of the brain via an *interrupt system*. (The use of interrupts is a style of computer programming in which one program is allowed to *interrupt* the processing of another program to communicate with it.) You can certainly see this happen in your own life: While you are in the middle of making lunch, you might pause for a minute because the cheese you are slicing reminds you of a bicycle picnic with your friend Lisa ten years ago, at which you ate cheese sandwiches while sitting beside a stream. Lisa was friends with *Gary*, and *Gary*, *Indiana*, was where the California guy (with the boat!), whose name you've been trying to remember, had family. So you stop making the cheese sandwiches for a moment—you get *interrupted* by the *try-to-remember-boat-guy's-name* daemon that has just jumped at its chance opportunity—because you now *almost* have boat-man's name. . . .

Thus, these background processes, or daemons, are an important part of human cognitive processing. And, it seems that the more typically intellectual one's life is—I am guessing associated also with a more high-functioning-personality lifestyle— the more important these background daemons become. In concussives, these processing daemons are negatively affected, sometimes dramatically, as follows:

Because daemons use up resources, a healthy brain regulates triggering them: it generally won't spawn a daemon unless that daemon is likely to do something useful, and it will put a cap on the number of daemons it will run simultaneously. But even in healthy brains this triggering process is not an exact, or even very conscious, process. You might, for example, get a song stuck in your head, and be driven by curiosity to play it over and over until you figure out what it is—even when you do not like the song, care about it, or care what its name is. A delicate balance exists between firing up daemons that might come up with something useful—following creative and heuristically intelligent "hunches"—and filtering out possible triggers that are not likely to lead to useful results.

This filtering process is an important part of intelligence, and of the efficient use of whatever native brainpower a person has at his disposal. If Gina fires up too few daemons, she'll be a dull, plodding sort of person who learns slowly, and only what is clearly directed by others. If she fires up just the right number, it will help her to be a witty, inquisitive, intuitive, creative sort of person who seems to make connections that others do not. If she fires up too many daemons, she will be a distracted, brain-fatigued, nonlinear, confused sort of person with all sorts of ideas that no one seems to "get," and which do not lead to much.

In concussives, the filtering process itself is affected. Inappropriate daemons are continually triggered, needlessly searching for meaning in unfiltered minutiae. Concussives' automatic sensory filters no longer work correctly, so the world has a tendency to become a nightmare of cognitive input that is "noticed," and thus must be *consciously* filtered: the sound of a truck driving down the road outside is given the same initial importance as the sound of a question from your daughter, sitting in front of you, with whom you are having a conversation:

Your daughter asks, "Hey Dad, have you seen my car keys?"

You are trying to parse the words, to separate them from the rest of the aural stream. A daemon has fired itself off and is looking for how the truck sound relates to the sound of the word *keys*: The truck is a *garbage* truck, which sounds like *garage*, which is where *cars* live. Cars have *keys*. This train of thought interferes with the understanding of your daughter's question. *Why would the keys be in the garage? Did I see her keys in the garage?*

A concussive also loses the ability for his daemons to interrupt other daemons in the middle of their processing. I myself experienced this frequently: the phenomena of realizing that I knew something, and *knowing* that I knew it, but not being able to use that information, while at the same time realizing that the conscious, focused part of my brain was in need of exactly that same information.*

Lastly—and very importantly—because low-level visual/spatial representations can be damaged in a concussive's brain, daemons may not realize, so to speak, that their conditions for termination have been met—the *match* against current circumstances fails—and they just keep running, well beyond their useful life.†

In each of these cases—spawning unneeded and unwanted daemons, being unable to solve problems because of a lack of information even though it may actually have already been

---

*I mentioned this in a talk, and afterward a recovered stroke victim told me I had precisely captured his own experience: he could hold a candy bar in his hand, and describe every aspect—and function—of it, but could not for the life of him tell you what it was, or himself make use of that information—even though he absolutely knew this in another part of his brain.

†In one fascinating episode, my respected Tai Chi teacher asked me to mail letters for him. I was having lots of trouble making sense of geometry at the time and could not "see" the *shape* of my having put the white rectangular envelopes *into* the opening in the mailbox. Thus the letter-mailing daemon did not recognize its termination conditions. I began to worry that an important letter did not get mailed for this esteemed master. Despite the fact that I *knew* full well that I had mailed the letters, I ended up calling my teacher repeatedly over the course of two weeks, describing the details (but not the gestalt) of my actions in placing the letters in the mailbox—asking if this was good enough—before the daemon finally resolved itself and went away. The link between daemon termination and *certainty* is thus also made clear.

located through another part of the brain's processing, and being unable to terminate daemons that have completed their tasks but can't form a visual/spatial pattern match to realize it—the result is that the brain grows increasingly fatigued, which in turn causes increasing difficulty with both sensory filtering and daemon communication, in a downward spiral of cognition failure.

From the outside, it just appears that a concussive is quirky and unreasonable about the noise of garbage trucks and the need for quiet in the household. He is slow in responding to simple questions about car keys, and asking such questions can make him unaccountably distressed. This does not make much sense to others, who are not aware of the processing overload that is going on under the hood.

You will often hear concussives complain that they "can only do one thing at a time." And this is true. The sad fact, however, is that normal cognition, even when only doing one thing at a time on the surface, often requires many layers of simultaneous processing in the brain.

DAEMON GUILT. Around this time, still in the early days after the accident, I had my first encounters with episodes of undifferentiated guilt: a guilt that crept up on me, and was triggered by subconscious processes, but which was not bound to any specific intentional actions I had taken. Such guilt feelings became quite common over the years.

Typically, I would be unsuccessfully trying to perform some task in my life—such as feeding myself during the apple-or-salami incident. I *knew* that I knew exactly how to perform the task, but I could not seem to access that knowledge of how to do it. At this point a "guilt daemon" would fire up, presumably to get me to stop screwing around and conform to societal conventions of handling my own problems, instead of acting so helplessly: after all, as far as the daemon was concerned, *all the knowledge to get the job done was available to me.*

I was left with this often-repeating circumstance where I knew how to act, knew what was to be done, felt guilty that I was not acting, but was powerless to initiate action toward my goals. But I was unable to make the guilt daemon "understand" that there was no way I could live up to the principle for which I was being held accountable. So, it would not go away, and actually made things worse by itself consuming precious resources.

Several years after the crash, Jake and I were leaving the Century Movie Theater in Evanston. Jake recognized that I was having some trouble walking—the parallel lines and moving planes on the long escalator ride down to the lobby were playing havoc with my highly vision-dependent balance systems. So, just as we were exiting through the glass doors of the theater, he said, "You can stay here if you want, and I'll go get the car."

Because of *cognitive slowing* (which we'll discuss in detail in a later section), one symptom of which was my inability to turn spoken sentences into meaning quickly enough to keep up with normal speech, I did not quite make out what he said. After some error correction, based on the few words I did get, and the overall sound of his utterance, I mistakenly thought Jake had said, "You can stay here if you want, and I'll try to make out what those are."

There were some pretty female Northwestern University grad students on the sidewalk to our left. As near as I could tell, Jake, an always-interested bachelor, was referring to the attractive women, although I couldn't figure out what his comment meant. I wondered what my staying by the door of the theater had to do with Jake and the students.

While I was thinking this over, I crossed the street with Jake, slowly walking alongside him, following him back toward the car. I looked toward the women and said, "I'm sorry, Jake, could you explain what you mean? I don't know how to decide if I should wait while you figure out what something is."

At exactly the time I started to speak, I also began to feel very distinctly guilty, which was unpleasant—a feeling of unnamed dread.

But this time, rather than deal with it on my own, I mentioned it to Jake. I was ready to look for some answers, and to analyze the details of what had just happened. Jake was game: scientific analysis of most any aspect of the natural world was something that he and I engaged in often. So we sat in his car and worked it out.

When Jake first spoke his sentence, I honestly did not hear all of the words clearly. This happens to all of us. Fortunately, however, most of us are almost instantaneously—and certainly without conscious thought—able to disambiguate an incorrectly heard utterance by replacing some words with others, so that the expressions make sense in the current circumstances: ". . . stay here if you want, and I will go get the car." In computer science terms this is simply a matter of meeting the constraints of the words that we *did* hear and those of the context in which we heard them, while searching for possible candidate-phrases with which to fill in the blanks, and then ranking our proposed solutions for viability. At some point one of the solutions is deemed *good enough* and we abandon further search.

However, my own ability to perform this kind of

constraint-based searching for the purposes of verbal stream error correction had been compromised, which is why certain kinds of conversations could make me very tired, very quickly. Yet this was a matter of degree: my error-correction processing was mostly still intact—just moving slowly.

Thus by the time I had determined the need for further information, formed the sentence that could request this information from Jake, and constructed the sounds necessary for uttering the question, a different part of my brain had already figured out what Jake had actually said.

Under the hood, so to speak, two daemons, S (*Search* for meaning) and Q (ask *Question*), had been started up, followed later by a third, G (*Guilt*). S was an independent *search daemon* whose job it was to find out the meaning of Jake's utterance. Failing to retrieve enough information to disambiguate the sentence on its own, S activated a *query daemon*, Q, to ask Jake to explain. But in the meantime, S kept searching. Because Q involved the forming of an utterance—a spoken sentence—it became the center of my attentional focus. That is, I was intentionally asking Jake a question; thus, everything else receded into the background, including the ongoing search by S for the error-corrected meaning of what Jake had originally said to me. In the middle of actually asking Jake the question, S had simultaneously figured out what Jake had said—obviating the need to ask the question at all.

Ordinarily this information from S would rise to the conscious level, and would abort the question-asking process, Q. But because of the brain damage, this communication from S to Q (and thus to my conscious level) could not take place. I still didn't "know" what Jake had said in any way I could make use of. For example, I couldn't make use of the information to stop walking, and tell Jake, "Thanks for your consideration. I'll wait for you here."

Meanwhile, under the surface, the preconditions for firing off a *guilt daemon* had been met: I was inconveniencing my friend, who was trying to help me. I was "pretending" not to have heard what he said. I was exacerbating my deceitfulness by now asking him to clarify his statement, even though I already knew the answer to my question. Each of these was a violation of one of my moral principles, and so an internal censure had been issued: guilt (G) rose of its own accord, independent of any conscious logic. I could not control it, and I could not make it go away.

It is interesting that whatever nonconscious process it was that triggered the guilt daemon (G) had access to both the process of my asking for information (Q), and the process that was reporting already having found that same information (S). But G did not have access to the abnormal structural constraint caused by the brain damage: while I had retrieved the missing information, *I could not access it* in any way that was useful to me. This makes sense, we might suppose. The first two processes are normal, and the guilt daemon is set up to handle them; but the guilt daemon was not designed to make use of a constraint solely caused by brain damage.

My intuition is that this had to do with what we will later understand were my ongoing difficulties with the integration of central attentional focus, and peripheral contextual information—important parts of the visual/spatial reasoning capabilities of the brain. In this case the detail/focus aspect of my interaction with Jake was my asking him questions about what he meant, and the peripheral context was that I had simultaneously already figured out what he had originally said.

Alas, guilt is not pleasant, especially when there is a feeling of having done something really bad but not knowing what it was. So this was a big moment for me—to understand why I had been feeling so guilty, so often, for two years, yet could never figure out how to "act right" so that I would not suffer from such relentless internal censuring. Our analysis allowed me to form a plan about this kind of recurring guilt such that, while it did not allow me to stop the emotion from occurring, it did allow me the solace of understanding what was happening to me: I could now ignore my guilt and simply shrug my shoulders in wonder at the marvelous design of the human mind.

BALANCE IN THE SYMBOLIC WORLD

Unless you have, yourself, lost efficacy in your balance system, you probably have no idea how devastating the effects of this can be in one's life. Because of inner-ear damage—yet another result of the crash—I had to deal with balance issues every day. In this section we'll start with the obvious challenges with basic motion for the concussive, but then must get progressively more sophisticated in our analysis as we examine the effects of balance difficulties on hearing, body sense, and even the most elemental aspect of cognition that make us human: the symbol creation of *thinking*.

THE THREE BALANCE SYSTEMS. Roughly speaking, the balance system uses three overlapping components: (a) the vestibular system, or "inner ear"; (b) the visual system; and (c) *proprioception*, the feeling of our bodies in the space around us—a position-movement sensation. While the vestibular system is primary, the other two are also very important, and the interaction among the three systems is far more complex than we generally consider.

Our vestibular and proprioceptive systems give direct information to our bodies to help them stay upright. But there is also a critical feedback loop between these two systems—processed in our brain stem—and our *eyes*. The *vestibulo-ocular reflex*, for example, takes input from the sensing of movement through neurological assessments of position and velocity and uses this information to stabilize our gaze by making micro-controlled adjustments in the *extraocular muscles* in the eyes so they counter head and body movements: the instant we move our head, our eyes adjust to stay fixed on an object. You can see this effect by looking directly at your own eyes in a mirror and moving your body around. In addition, these subsecond microadjustments are integrated with our ability to simultaneously adjust for the *pursuit* of objects moving in our environment as well, so we can turn our heads and bodies while still following the path of a bird flying across our yard. So our balance system controls our eyes.

But the relationship between our eyes and our balance system works in the other direction as well, and our *eyes control our balance*: when our vestibular system is underfunctioning—as often happens with head injury—our eyes can take over much of the load. We can illustrate this with a simple exercise: (1) Stand on one leg with your eyes open and your other knee up high—usually this is not too much of a problem. Notice the muscle adjustments in the foot that is on the floor. (2) Close your eyes, but continue standing on the one leg. Depending on how effective your vestibular and proprioceptive systems are, you will experience varying degrees of increased difficulty when losing your visual input (and a corresponding increase in the microadjustments in your foot). The more your balance is dependent on your vision system, the more you'll start to wobble when you close your eyes.

MOTION DISORIENTATION. Like many concussives, I had many episodes involving motion sickness that gave me trouble. For example, several weeks after the crash I tried to take the El train downtown. Within a few stops I was so sick that I vomited in the train car and had to roll myself out through the doors onto a platform.

"I'm sorry!" I said to the variously disgusted and concerned passengers. "I don't know what happened. I'm sorry." It took me three hours to recover sufficiently before I could walk home.

On an evening almost a year later, I was exhausted from teaching class and it was hard for me to walk—it had taken me an hour to get down the stairs of the classroom building. I didn't want to face walking up the stairs again in the building where my office was, so I talked myself into thinking it would be okay to take the elevator up to the sixth floor. This was a mistake. Once the elevator doors opened on six, I tumbled out onto the floor and crawled to the wall, where I could prop myself up. I rested there for fifteen minutes, pretending to be sitting on the floor reading a book whenever students came by. Then I crawled to my office on my hands and knees, and rested on the floor for an hour to recover my equilibrium.

We'll see later that because of the strong link between our balance systems and our eyes, it is possible that many people who suffer from what they assume to be congenital motion sickness would improve by treating their *visual* systems.

BALANCE, VISION, AND THOUGHT.* Because I had suffered vestibular system damage, this meant that my already-overtaxed and poorly functioning visual system had to take on the additional load of providing for many of my balance needs as well. But at the same time, any sort of high-level thinking also required the use of exactly those same visual/spatial systems in creating the internal *images* of thought.

Thus we have the following: Under the *cognitive load of thinking*—which almost always entailed visualization, pattern matching, and generating the spatial imagery to form analogies— my damaged brain would rapidly grow fatigued. The visual/spatial circuitry would get overloaded, and could no longer manage its double-duty making up for the vestibular system, and I would *lose my balance.* As we will see, the same thing would happen when I had to use my visual/spatial circuitry to interpret *meaning* in complex sensory input—such as speech, or the complicated visual patterns on store shelves. One of the worst combinations would be when I had to use the visual systems in my brain simultaneously for both complex thinking, or sensory interpretation, *and* intense balance calculations.

As my brain fatigue grew during even short periods of cognitive load my balance would grow progressively worse, and nausea would almost immediately set in. Depending on

---

*Because my experience with this was so ubiquitous, and so debilitating, I consider it to be one of the most crucial concepts we will consider, and perhaps one of the most helpful for those with TBI.

what I was thinking about, or the physical task I was working on, I would start to lose my balance within five minutes.

I developed a surreptitious remedial balance technique: whenever I walked around the university—where I had to *think* throughout the day—I would simply run an index finger along a wall as though I were goofing around. People tended not to notice this much, especially if I kept my hand low on the wall, and it was much better than looking drunk by weaving around in hallways and classrooms.

A neurological oddity that presented itself in my case, and that you might notice in a concussive who is having balance problems, was that my index fingers would flex upward, with my thumbs out-thrust, while the rest of my fingers were re-laxed downward, forming a flexed "L" between the thumb and index finger of each hand. If you put your arms out at slightly less than a forty-five-degree angle and raise your index fingers in this way, you will likely perceive this as a kind of balance-vigilant position.

WHERE THE BODY ENDS. Our balance systems are integrated with other important but little-considered systems as well. For example, a collection of nerves in the superior parietal lobe is thought to help us distinguish where our bodies end and where the external world takes over. Without the capability to make this distinction, it would be difficult for us to navigate our way through a world filled alternately with obstructions and openings through them. At times, brain activity in this area is naturally reduced and our sense of where our bodies end is appropriately minimized—for example, when we drop off to sleep, or fall into a deep meditative state.

This body-demarcation sense is something that normals

take for granted, but it can be quite troubling when it disappears at unnatural times. It is an interesting question to consider the relationships among the brain's visual cortex, our balance systems, and this body-versus-surroundings demarcation sense. My experience suggests that there is a link. Under brain stress—primarily visual, and especially when making excessive demands on my visual system for balance—the boundary line between my body and the rest of the world became blurred.

This was most easily noticed in my almost ubiquitous (though relatively mild) difficulty passing through doorways, down tunnels (such as stairways and Jetways), and getting into cars, when my brain was tired. I would have to put my arms out to "feel" the spatialness of the opening—using my eyes to carefully examine the distinctions between my hands and the surrounding objects—and thus guide myself through manually.

A more striking example of this loss of body-environment demarcation occurred five years after the crash, as a result of a set of intense visual-balance demands:

One of the fifty-foot trees in my back yard had been identified as having Dutch elm disease, which can spread throughout a neighborhood, so it had to be cut down. High-ladder tree work of this kind is intense, and not for the faint of heart. I couldn't afford to have it professionally removed, so in the end I had to manage it on my own.*

I knew I would have to contend not only with the normal rather striking visceral reactions of being so high up, but also

---

*To set this in context, consider that a pair of super-macho day laborers who had earlier done heavy work on the foundation of my house showed up and said they would cut the tree down for a budget price. They laughed and taunted each other before climbing up to get to work, but each of them returned down the ladder after only a minute—with their knees uncontrollably shaking. They soon gave up, and left.

with the added complications from my brain damage. The following diary passage is from a day when I had climbed thirty feet into the tree to cut off the highest branches, which themselves reached another twenty feet over my head. This episode simultaneously taxed my visual/spatial system for three separate tasks: the intense spatial planning of where the heavy tree branches were to be cut, and would fall; the meaningful interpretation of the incoming barrage of sensory input; and the essential need to keep my balance based primarily on the constantly moving visual input.

I am disoriented because I can't look down, and so have to get my visual bearings from watching parts of the tree, which are themselves swaying in the wind. It's all one chaotic swirl of sunlit green. My balance system is shot, and I have to rely on my eyes only to know which way is up. The flood of data from my senses is overwhelming: the roar from the chainsaw engine; the smell of oil burning on the muffler; the feel of branches pressing against me everywhere; sawdust, salty sweat, and stinging two-stroke exhaust in my eyes and that I taste in my mouth. I am having difficulty managing the *geometry* of placing myself—my body, and the chainsaw I'm holding—within the context of the moving tree. It's as though I've lost my sense of the demarcation point of—the boundary between—my inner self and the outer world around me. Except for what my eyes can tell me as I stare intensely through the fog of my safety glasses at both my boot, and the saw ripping through the branch on which that boot is standing, I have no way of distinguishing between the two. I have to manually, continually, walk myself through the connections in the branching of the tree, and the differential branching of my body. I can't tell the difference between the two. Terrifying—given the circumstances, but also fascinating . . .

It goes without saying that after I climbed down I was unable to walk, or even to stand up. Having to manage the chainsaw without the natural protection of knowing where my body ended was intense, and the base fear this truly odd experience generated was extreme. It took me a week to get the tree down, and another two weeks after that before my brain recovered.

BALANCE AND HEARING. Balance is also linked indirectly to our aural processing systems because most of us process the meaning of audio input in a visual/symbolic way, and this in turn can compete with the visual processing needed for balance.

An extreme illustration of this can be found in my notes from August, two years after the crash. I was driving back east with my friend James to attend my aunt's funeral, and to visit James's relatives in Maine. Even though James knew me well, like so many others he didn't "get" that there was anything really wrong with me. James wanted to do all the driving, and traveling as a passenger in his car was a challenge. I had to keep my eyes continually focused on the horizon to help keep my equilibrium.

James liked listening to the news on the radio, but this was a problem for me: I was unable to filter out the talk-audio stream, which meant that my visual system was being used—regardless of whether I wanted it to be—to create images of scenes from the radio news. This in turn meant that my visual system was unavailable to be used for balance, and I started to become both nauseated and disoriented. I managed to get by, sort of, until evening, but it took a heavy toll on me. My deep batteries were drained.

When it grew dark, the problem got worse because the distant horizon was no longer available for me to use for keeping my balance. And James had to have the radio on to help him stay awake.

We decided to stop driving for the night, but unfortunately we were unable to find a motel room. It seems that this was peak season for paintball, Mohican powwows, car shows, and other summer attractions in Indiana and Ohio. James grew increasingly fatigued, and frustrated, and began to whip the car around corners at each interstate exit as we tried over and over again to find a place to stay.

This violent motion of the car, combined with the extreme fatigue of my visual systems, and especially the processing demands from the car radio audio stream, made it impossible for me to keep my balance, and in the end put me over the edge. I asked James to stop the car, but he thought I was just being difficult. So at midnight, at a stoplight, a mile away from the most recent interstate exit we had taken, I poured myself out of the car and into the street. There was a brief conversation about money in my pocket, which I didn't understand, and then James drove off. I crawled over to a grassy patch under a lighted billboard, next to a truck-repair parking lot.

From the environment, I knew that I was in a seedy part of a decaying midwestern industrial town in the middle of the night. Other than that I had no idea where I was, how I got there, or even *who I was*. I just needed the world to stop spinning inside of me, and outside of me. I needed the bell of nausea in which I was living to open and let me out. I stared up at the billboard, and the city lights reflecting off the cloudy sky above it, unable to comprehend anything at all.

An hour later, James, relenting, came back to get me. He had found a motel. After we drove there, he went up to the room and went to sleep, leaving me alone to arrange my own belongings. I sat on the curb next to the car, without the slightest clue about how to proceed. A gang of toughs came by, carrying bottles of liquor in paper bags. They jeered at me, shoving me with their feet. I thought they might steal my things, or beat me up, but in the end they left. It took me an hour of intense work to get from the car to room 201, which was only fifty feet away, guiding myself through the chaos one inch at a time. I inched my way up the stairs and into the room, then fell asleep on the floor with my eyes open.

BALANCE AS A COMPONENT OF THOUGHT. It is seldom considered, but in fact balance is linked to basic cognition, and is part of the way we construct multifaceted symbols in our brain. Without the orienting-within-space grounding of the balance system it becomes almost impossible to think clearly. When I lost my own sense of balance during times of brain distress, I also coincidentally found that the symbols I used for all kinds of problem solving became impoverished as well.

For example, we think of the concept of a *symmetric relationship* as being "the same in each direction." But the subconcept of *direction*, at least for me, includes as part of it a sense of space, a sense of objects being present in that space, and the idea of potential motion from one of the objects to the other.

With symmetry, whatever "happens to" one of the objects also "happens to" the other object, albeit in a reversed direction. But each of these images—direction, space, objects in space, motion, "happens to," and reversal—in turn tends to involve the even more basic concept of a horizon, and upness and downness, and leftness and rightness as well, each grounded in our *balanced orientation in the world.*

Furthermore, these thought-objects are placed in space, often in front of our foreheads, certainly not behind our ears or our knees, so our own orientation within the thinking landscape is part of our reference. When the balance system is malfunctioning, essential elements (our perspective, orientation in space, "leftness," "upness," etc.) of each of these basic features ("happens to," direction, motion, etc.) of the basic symbols of thought (symmetry, relationship, etc.) leave us. We can still think, and still manipulate symbols, but once again the visual system has to overfunction to make up for the absent natural richness of the original symbols. This is very fatiguing, and often not maintainable for more than a few minutes.*

Maintaining balance in our lives goes far beyond merely staying upright.

---

*One of my graduate students—who also had suffered a brain injury—said that he understood *exactly* about the loss of elemental cognitive concepts when he had balance problems. In his case the most pronounced result was a flattening of affect, because he could not support the concepts of complex emotions without the more basic concepts of relationship between himself and others, and between himself and the world.

VISUAL/SPATIAL PATTERNS, SHAPES, RELATIONSHIPS

WHEN GEOMETRY LOSES ITS STRUCTURE. In the few months prior to the crash, I had started to gut the burned house I was living in, so that I could rebuild it. I had four brick walls, three doors, and a few newly replaced windows, as my home. I was using a duct-taped garden hose and a laundry tub for a shower, and most important—with the Chicago winter looming—I was soon to have no roof. It was unfortunate that it was at this point in the rebuilding process that I got the concussion.

Because funds were so extremely dear, I felt I had no choice but to continue with the rebuilding, working with subcontractors and doing much of the work myself. But this meant that with almost no ability to form or understand plans, I still had to be on the job every day managing all aspects of this large project.

I did virtually all of the shopping for parts and supplies

myself. On a typical shopping day, I might arrive at Home Depot with a list of a hundred complicated parts that the plumber needed *that day* in order to keep working: twelve 60° angled male-to-female ¾ inch PVC joints, four ¾ inch copper sweat-fit right-angle joints, an inverted water-tank pressure-relief valve, and so on.

Scanning for items in a store is a highly structured visual process that makes use of much conceptual information in the brain to rapidly interpret the massive amounts of visual data coming in. The data is sorted and filtered according to the concepts: horizontal shelves, and the vertical stacking of those shelves; shelves arranged in bays; the bays in aisles; the aisles in departments. The objects on the shelves have sizes, shapes, and colors, and these are used to index and chunk together the store items in an organized way.

For example, if you see a can of Glidden latex paint, which has an easily identifiable Glidden label, and your peripheral vision indicates that all the other objects on the same horizontal plane have the same labels, the same colors, the same sizes, and the same shapes, then there is an immediate, visceral understanding that this is a shelf full of *Glidden paint*. If you are looking for Behr paint, whose cans have the same shape as Glidden cans, but differently colored labels, or are looking for plumbing parts, which have a different shape entirely from that of paint cans, then a normal brain will immediately, through a low-level visual-symbolic process, remove all bays containing Glidden paint from the search. It is not necessary to look at *each* can of paint and try to decide if it is the object you are looking for.

With the kind of visual disturbance I suffered, searching for my plumbing parts soon deteriorated into a process that can be imagined as follows:

Take all four thousand objects that will pass across your field of vision when walking through the plumbing aisle and randomly place them in a large patch of open floor. Take the cardboard tubes from the middle of a pair of paper-towel rolls and tape them over your eyes so that you can only see what is directly in the center of your field of vision, and so that what you are seeing has no peripheral context at all. Now, for the first item on your shopping list, start walking through the store items that are randomly placed on the floor. For each object on the floor, pick it up, and without naming it, describe the *details* of it to your brain to see whether it matches the first item on your list, which you are now trying to find: the color, the shape, the corners, the texture, its mass, and any interesting features it might have. Taken all together, do these features constitute the *PVC elbow joint* that you are looking for? If so, then try to locate your cart and put the elbow joint in it. Otherwise, put it back on the floor. Having located the first item on your list in this way, move on to the next one.

Note that in walking through the four thousand items that are strewn about the floor there is no way to recognize whether you have returned to some spot you have already visited. There is no global field of vision. And, too, there are only the tiny component features (e.g., color, texture, angles) that make up the objects themselves: you've lost the ability to automatically translate these features of the objects into the gestalt of the "thing" itself.

As you grow more brain-fatigued, the tubes over your eyes get smaller in diameter, and your ability to describe the features of the items to your brain deteriorates as well. You move ever more slowly. At some point what's known as *thrashing* sets in: you are taking so long to examine any one object that by the time you have gotten around to describing the last of its features to your brain, you have forgotten what the first features were, and you have to go back to refresh that part of your description—in an endless loop. Ultimately, you have to stop.

This is what it is like to go shopping for plumbing parts when you have concussion brain damage.

After five minutes of searching through shelves and bins, my head would start to hurt. After ten minutes I would have to hold on to the shelving to stand up. In twenty minutes the nausea would be problematic. After thirty minutes I would be almost completely unable to make sense of the visual scene, apprehending only the component features of items directly in front of me, in the center of my vision: a bit of texture, some color, a shadowing, an angle formed by the joining of two edges, and so on.

By this point I would lose the spatial sense of being "in an aisle" in the store. I would lose all concept of horizontal space, and could no longer see "shelfness." I was moving in slow motion. I had to support myself by holding on to the shopping cart if I moved down the aisle.

Sometimes I could find a plumbing associate in the store who would help me find some of the parts. But this was tricky. If I asked them where to find an "inverter plate," which was written down on my list but not something with which I was familiar, it might turn out that it was right in front of me. But if the associate said, "It's right there next to the green shutoff valves on the top shelf," it could be trouble. I couldn't rapidly retrieve the concepts of "shelf," "top," and "green," and what a valve looked like (*valves? valve?—circular motion* . . . , *piston* . . . , *tubelike object* . . . ?). I would typically say something like, "I'm really sorry, but I don't have my correct glasses on, and can't see very well. Could you point to it?" But I did not *look* like a person who could not see. After pointing out two or three items, associates would get impatient with my slowness and drift off to help other customers.

At some point I would give up and head for the checkout counter, doing my best to appear normal. Several times, early on, I pushed myself too far, and had to leave my cart in an aisle and go to my car to rest. The sensory overload from the unfiltered sights and sounds was too much for me.

Lines at the checkout counter could also be problematic; once my body stopped moving I would get stuck, resting my head on the shopping cart and unable to move forward when a gap opened up. It was difficult to understand speech. If the cashier asked any questions about an item ("Is this washer galvanized?"), I just had them put it back, saying, "I'm very sorry. I don't want it now." Over time I learned how to push myself just far enough that I could still pay for my items, find my car, and get home.

After checkout came what was often the most difficult part of a shopping trip, especially if it was during the winter and cold: finding my car in the parking lot.

I would stand by the exit doors, not having a clue where my car was, not able to get my legs to move, viewing the world as though everything were a mile away. I could make no sense of the spatial characteristics of parking lots after shopping: the grids, the compass orientation, the parking aisles, the colors and shapes of the cars. And because my memory of where I had parked the car was stored using these low-level concepts, I had no idea where to look for it. I might wander around a parking lot for half an hour, examining the minute details of each car as I came up next to it, trying to decide whether it was mine. In the winter I was often freezing by the time I found my car. Then I had to wait a long time before my brain settled and I knew it was safe to drive.

I often thought longingly about those handicap parking spaces near the entrance of the store. Having a handicap sticker would have been such a godsend! But government regulations did not make allowances for a long-distance runner who was yet often unable to walk to navigate a parking lot after shopping.*

NORTH SOUTH EAST WEST. You will recall that on the day of the accident I had trouble navigating to the police station to retrieve my driver's license. Within a few days I realized that I'd completely lost my sense of direction, which had always been grounded in the North-South-East-West (NSEW) grid that can be laid over the earth. My former sense of direction had been so acute that I had once intuitively retraced my steps for fifteen miles, through entirely urban terrain, to a house in an obscure and anonymous neighborhood full of curving streets, which I had visited exactly once—when buying a car from a stranger five years earlier.†

---

*Ultimately, after five years one M.D. did go out on a limb and say, "Sure, of course," and sign a form for me. The rest of the paperwork took me a difficult month to get through; the rearview-mirror placard was only good for three months; much of the time the Chicago Police ignored the placard and gave me a ticket anyway. It was great at Home Depot, but the paperwork was far too exhausting to ever apply for a *temporary* placard again.

†This sense of direction is represented as a spectrum in the general population and is also thought to be at least somewhat sex-linked, relating to—and here relevant to our discussion—*spatial rotation* capabilities.

By contrast, my friend Jake had no NSEW grounding whatsoever. Before my concussion, our contrasting styles of navigation used to clash when traveling: Jake had a Garmin GPS device in his car, and always set it so that maps were displayed with north pointing *up*. This drove me out of my mind, and if I wore Jake down enough he'd relent and finally let me set the Garmin so that north pointed *north*. Similarly, if we had a map laid out on a table, Jake would set the map so north was facing up, away from him, but I would always turn the map so that it corresponded to the real face of the earth—even if it meant I was reading the words upside down. At a visceral level it was hard for me to imagine always being as lost in the world as Jake seemed, to me, to be.

When I lost my "perfect direction" sense in the moment of the crash, I lost all of my absolute grounding in the directional-symbolic world as well. This loss is much more profound than simply having to relearn how to get around the city, using a map. I found that many of the basic symbols of my intellectual-mathematical life had also been grounded in my directional sense, and having lost *it* I also lost important parts of *them*. Thus I lost foundational, elemental pieces that gave meaning to numbers, relations, analogies, and functions. I could no longer, for example, "see" the number seven in the same way, and when I tried to use it in even simple arithmetical calculations, I struggled. For me, the number seven had always in some obscure way stretched *east*, a component concept that no longer had any internal meaning.

I also had trouble with dreams. Ordinarily, it was my experience that dreams helped me work out—in a highly symbolic way—ongoing problems that arose during my waking life. But for me the linking between the two worlds—dream and real—was highly spatial in nature, including *directionally* spatial. That is, formerly the concept of "north" actually *was* north—in my dreams and in the real world—and this was an important linkage between the two. In this way, for example, some dream-vision of a long green-lit corridor with a red-striped carpet, and through which I was walking, would *of course* be oriented northeast/southwest, because my conception of the corresponding real-world difficulty was also oriented in that diagonal way on the face of the earth—say representing a conflict between two friends whose houses lay in that particular northeast/southwest orientation. Although I continued to have the same types of shape- and relationship-filled dreams, I would wake up with the distinct feeling that they had taken place in a groundless, disoriented world, and could no longer be linked to real life in a way that carried meaning. Thus my dreams were often no longer productive in the same way. I'd lost the *perfect reference* in which I could work out problems.

But how hard this is to explain to a normal! There is no checkbox on a neurologist's form, nor is there a *DSM-5* code to describe this unsettling loss. "Doctor, do you have a diagnosis for me? I can't find north in my dreams anymore. . . ."

SLEEP AND THE VISUAL SYSTEM. In addition to losing the NSEW grounding of my dreams, I had other visual/spatial problems associated with sleep, some of them surprising.

In previous passages we have seen that I learned to fall asleep with my eyes open, and in the first few months after the crash I had to resort to this often to keep from getting seasick once I closed my eyes. But sleeping with one's eyes open is not necessarily so unusual. Some parents reading this may recall those times when they've checked on their babies at night wondering if they have a zombie child: sound asleep, staring sightlessly off into the distance.

Contemporary research, indicated by self-reporting but consistent with fMRI scans, suggests that people vary widely in how "visual" they are in their thinking. Some people create images in their minds that are almost as vivid as the deepest, most vivid dreams. A small percentage of the population reports not being visual at all in their thinking. I am toward the high end of the spectrum of visual thinkers. I made use of this predilection, for example, in my graduate study days, when I actively trained myself to enter a mild "lucid dreaming" state when working on the most difficult problems.

Similarly, there is a wide range in how much people dream. The conventional thinking has long been that people dream during REM sleep, and experience dreamless sleep at other times. But it turns out that some people also dream during the non-REM periods, and this is only sometimes associated with disorders. Prior to the crash I was at the absolute end of the bell curve of sleep dreamers: if I was asleep I was dreaming. Always.*

My being a highly visual thinker, combined with the fact that if I was asleep I was dreaming, happened to be two parts of an unfortunately bad mix, especially during the first year after the crash. By the end of the day, the visual processing

---

*Interestingly, after treatment, I am now more toward the center: I have periods of both dreaming and dreamless sleep. Some people who dream all the time wake up perpetually tired (see, e.g., "epic dream disorder") and we have to wonder if the kinds of treatment I received might also help them. Further evidence to suggest this might be worth pursuing is the number of such people who also report balance problems.

parts of my brain were almost always exhausted, and were what most needed rest. But dreaming is primarily a *visual* exercise—especially so for a highly visual thinker like me. This meant that during the process of falling asleep I would immediately enter into my visually vivid dream world, and within a few minutes would become exhausted, nauseated, and completely disoriented—absolutely overwhelmed. When I was in this state, instead of going to sleep, no matter how tired I was, I had to sit and stare at some object five to ten feet away, doing absolutely nothing that would require the creation of any scenes in my head—any of the symbols of thought. (And although I didn't piece it together until later, it turned out that on days when I did not have to make too much use of my eyes for balance, I could often sleep in the normal way.)

After an hour or two, or four, or six, of sitting there being completely, staggeringly bored, my brain was rested enough to support the imagery of dreaming, and I could allow myself to fall asleep.

One of the other sleep symptoms I began to experience one or two times a month after the crash was *sleep paralysis*—a startling state in which I would wake up enough to rise into consciousness, with full sentient awareness of my body, but was not awake enough to be able to move at all, in what is known as *complete REM paralysis.**

The most disconcerting problem of sleep paralysis, and

---

*Many people who experience sleep paralysis at one point or another also have hypnagogic hallucinations—embodied as visions of various demon incubi or succubi sitting on their legs, or whispering in their ears, and so on. Given the already somewhat terrifying nature of sleep paralysis, I have to say I am *extremely* glad I never experienced these latter symptoms!

one often experienced immediately upon waking in this eerie state, is that your natural inclination will be to take a deep breath in anticipation of the need for action, but because of the paralysis nothing happens. Your body, which is still asleep, is in fact autonomously getting enough air for its needs, but it *feels* like you are suffocating, since you're not consciously able to draw breath. You might also experience other minor bodily discomforts, suddenly magnified in a claustrophobic way because you can't do anything about them: you might feel too hot, or your limbs might be uncomfortable, but it's impossible to move. Finally, with great effort, after a few long minutes have passed, you can usually move an eyelid, or a fingertip, and, as with the initiation problem, this gives enough feedback to get the body moving again. You can finally breathe in a gasping lungful of air.

I find it troubling that so many people (reportedly, many millions of people) have to deal with sleep paralysis, and it is often considered exclusively from a psychiatric perspective as part of a general category of sleep disorders. The fact is, I never had this problem before the crash. I suffered from it for the eight years following the crash. I got better after effective treatment for concussion, and I've never had it again. Doesn't this at least suggest the possibility that people who suffer from this frightening condition might benefit from the same sort of primarily visual-system treatments that we'll later see I received?

We also might be suspicious that at least some of those who suffer from sleep paralysis may have had earlier, undiagnosed brain concussions. In my own family, the one of my children who suffered regularly from sleep paralysis was also the one who had incurred a serious concussion from a bicycle fall.

Because of my eight years' experience on the other side, so to speak, I now have a lifelong appreciation of the graceful way that most of us can slip so elegantly into and out of sleep, and the natural effortlessness with which this complex transition is managed.

RELATIONSHIP IN MEDITATION. When considering the long hours I spent being painfully bored, staring at a wall, doing nothing, giving my visual system a rest, a reasonable person might ask, what about meditation? After all, one of the goals of many kinds of meditation is embracing nothingness: being so present in the current moment that you are doing nothing at all. This seems ideal for giving visual systems in the brain a rest, while also using the time in a productive, self-enhancing, and restorative way. Alas, these two forms of nothingness—the type I pursued when trying to rest my concussion-wearied brain, and the kind pursued by meditators—are very different, in important ways.

Prior to the crash, at times of great intellectual demand, I found that I could rest in a meditative state and would emerge rejuvenated. An hour's focused meditation would be equivalent to several hours' worth of sleep.

Sometimes I would meditate in traditional ways. More often I would listen to music late at night, and would enter into a deeply meditative state, fully awake, without thought, highly concentrated, seeing nothing but a real-time vision of the music unfolding before my closed eyes. I would "see" the sounds of the music as interacting colors and shapes in all their interwoven complexity. It was pure sensory input, without thought. If someone spoke to me during such a meditation I wouldn't be able to hear her, as though I were in a deep sleep. I tuned out the sound of voices just as I tuned out acoustic defects in the recordings. But if my interrupter became more intrusive, such as by tapping me on the shoulder, I might startle awake, even involuntarily calling out as I was wrenched back up from those deep levels of concentration.

Meditation, and to my mind at least, every contemplative practice, has the critical element of *relationship*. Such states are experienced as a profound unveiling of the relationship of the individual to the rest of the universe, a revealing of the interconnectedness of life, and spirit, and the world. It is a becoming of the moment, and an understanding of how that moment is connected to all other moments both prior and following.

But all of this, the sense of relationship to God, the spiritual connection to the universe, and the global sense of nothingness/everythingness, is *highly visual/spatial in nature*. It was unequivocally my experience that I could not enter into such a state without making use of the spatial processing areas of my brain. And of course, this was exactly the part of my brain that so often needed rest.

For this reason, meditation was not often something I could engage in after the crash, and was most especially one of the worst things I could do when my visual systems were debilitated.

DIALOGUE WITH GOD AND THE MATTER OF SENTIENCE. Since my very early teens, I've had the sense of a dialogue with God. Though I did not grow up religious, praying was easy for me. I talked to God, and God listened. God talked to me (in pictures, and through intuition), and I listened. Dialogue with the spirit was easy and natural: comforting, occasionally demanding, *real*.

Almost immediately following the crash, this dialogue disappeared. I recall very distinctly entering the small chapel at

DePaul's downtown university campus, sitting alone on one of the chairs to pray for my students, and for my ability to serve them as their professor—something I often did. In a profoundly disturbing moment I realized that there was no longer anyone there. No one was listening. I thought: *These are just empty words I am saying to myself. My prayers are no different than if I were reading aloud from an auto repair manual.*

I felt a deep sense of loss, but in a weird way. Though I understood, intellectually, about the loss of dialogue with God, and I felt quite disturbed about how sterile my life had become because of it, I nonetheless couldn't quite "see" what was missing. It was like trying to remember a dream. I still believed in God, but viscerally it was an entirely different experience: there was no longer anyone there.

When we consider the nature of my later recovery, and the many examples we've seen of how our internal world is so very symbolic in nature, it becomes apparent that it was the loss of my visual/spatial ability to represent symbolic *relationship* that was at the heart of my troubles with God. If so, then losing the closeness to God I felt pre-concussion raises some interesting questions about our connection to the larger universe around us. Could this sense of connection be located entirely in one of the visual/spatial centers of our brains? After all, in my case I had this easy faith up until the moment of the crash. I lost it in the days after the crash. I didn't have it for eight years. I got it back again after treatment for my concussion. This is pretty strong evidence that it is our brains—our *physical* brains—that support this kind of spiritual faith.

What this means is still up for grabs, however. As scientists, we have to allow for at least two possibilities. On the one hand we could take this as evidence that a sense of God, and the spirit, is just an artifact of the neural, and possibly other, programming in our brains—a purely physical uprising from a locus in our heads. Certainly there are researchers who talk about the "God spot" in the parietal, and other, regions of the brain that are thought to give rise to spirituality. Some have even have claimed to have created a "God Helmet" that artificially stimulates a profound religious experience via artificial manipulation of the brain.* On the other hand, we could just as easily imagine that these parts of the brain allow us to connect to a real channel of spirituality, and that without them we have simply lost one dimension of our sensory capabilities. That is, if we lose our hearing, the world is still full of sound; in the same way, if we lose our sense of God, that doesn't mean that God is not still out there.

There is another, related question that we have already raised: we have discussed that concussives often feel as though they have become nonhuman. In my case I felt this profoundly. And, as we will see, when the Ghost later returns, it is because my brain can once again support the *necessary cognition* for being fully human. So what does this tell us about the nature of any sort of life after death? No one will disagree that our brains are physical devices, and that they perform all sorts of computational functions on our behalf. If losing some of the brain's computational capabilities causes us to become so very much less human, then what does this say about our humanness when the physical brain stops functioning altogether? After all, we don't take our brains with us when we die.

---

*Reported by inventor Stanley Koren and neuroscientist Michael Persinger, though others have not been able to replicate their results. Regardless, *neuroethology*—the study of such phenomena—is an ongoing branch of research.

A scientist might then suspect that life after death—life without a physical brain—might necessarily be a very foreign, thoroughly nonhuman existence indeed.

These are not trivial questions. As computers get increasingly powerful, most thoughtful cognitive scientists must take such questions seriously. Consider the following enigma:

Suppose we built a synthesized mind, which runs on a computer. It is completely artificial, and there is no part of it that is not implemented as zeros and ones in silicon registers. Most of us would have no problem terminating the artificial mind by turning off the computer, or frightening it, because we know it is not real. It doesn't *actually* feel anything—after all, we are just, say, replacing a "0001" with a "0011" in some *fear register*. On the other hand, those of us who are not sociopaths *would* have a problem terminating the gardener working next door, or frightening him, because he has a right to life, and *does* feel the emotional pain of being scared. One is real, the other is not.

Yet we can imagine that in the coming years we will be building very much more complex artificial minds—ultimately, perhaps as complex as those of humans. But they are still artificial, right? Because they are running as zeros and ones on silicon chips . . .

Not so fast. If both the computer and the human are simply computational devices—software activations of zeros and ones running on silicon hardware in one case, and neural activations running on a brain and body system in the other—then what about the following:

From a theoretical standpoint, we can fully implement all the functions of a single neuron (or glial cell, etc.) with a modern computer. We can model all its input and output functions, and also all its networked connections to other neurons. So now, one by one, we replace each brain cell of our gardener working next door with a networked computer that fully implements both that cell and all of its connections to other cells. At some point, we will have replaced *all* of the gardener's brain cells with our exact artificial copies of them. We have turned our gardener into a computer, but one that *fully implements him*. (Keep in mind that every thought, every memory, every feeling—including the most minute aspect of our gardener's sense of self—would be supported in either case—human or computer—and in every hybrid case along the way.)*

Because the gardener's mind and the computer-simulated mind each can be transformed into the other, at what point is the gardener real, and at what point artificial? Do we simply argue that there is some "critical mass" of complexity after which sentience arises within *any* such system, regardless of the implementation? With the advent of computer science, issues such as the dualism arguments of Descartes and Ryle become grounded in precision: when we build a computer model, each bit is on, or it is off, completely, irrefutably, implementing the minutest part of our theory.

And what happens, then, when we build such systems from scratch? Do *they* have rights? The right to "life"? Does it now become unethical for us to turn them off? Do they, independently of us, communicate with God?

Or, suppose that separate from the ability to build artificial life in this way, we also have the ability to manipulate its

---

*And of course we could, in theory, also reverse the process—turning our computer brain into a human one by replacing our computer implementations with the real cells they are modeling, one by one. Each of these is a variation of what is known as the "China brain" conundrum discussed by Lawrence Davis in 1974.

configuration. Suppose that, having isolated the computational (feeling of?) connection to God that I lost for eight years, we can build artificial beings that always experience this connection, and are in a constant state of enlightened bliss. Are we then obligated to build as many of them as we can, in the way that we feel obligated to do our best so that our children have happy, possibly spirit-based lives?

These are interesting questions, not so easily answered, but also, in the computer age, not so easily dismissed. And my own experience—my partial loss of human sentience coinciding with my loss of brain functionality—brought them *much* closer to home.

TIME IS A METAPHOR

WHEN TIME LOSES ITS STRUCTURE. In 2001, two years after the crash, I went to see the recently released movie *Memento*, a drama with an odd narrative structure in which time runs both forward and backward in a series of flashbacks and "flash-forwards." The main character, Leonard, suffers from short-term memory loss and can only remember recent events for a few minutes. In trying to unravel a rapist-drug-dealer murder mystery and find his wife's killer, he records important events by tattooing summaries of them on his body so he won't forget them.

I hadn't known anything about the movie prior to entering the theater—a rare opportunity had arisen for some time off, and I'd simply picked a movie at random. After just the first few scenes I was sickened by what I was seeing, but mesmerized nonetheless. The director, Christopher Nolan, had managed to capture so clearly the *essence* of what I was going through every day of my life. I was both horrified to see so clearly in front of me what my life was like, and how truly incapacitated I was, but also, at the same time, grateful that at least one central truth of my existence could be captured and expressed.

Unlike the main character in *Memento*, I did not have short-term memory loss. Nor did I have to tattoo events on my body to remember them. And, of course, I was not trying to find the murderers of my wife. So why did this movie have such a strong, sad, remorseful, cathartic, essence-capturing effect on me?

For concussives, there is a disturbance in the normal apprehension of *time*. Most people in the Western world have an innate sense of time flowing smoothly, endlessly, from the past, through the present, and into the future. At least, this is how we Westerners *talk* about time, and conceptualize it when making plans and explaining our lives. But concussives can lose this (seemingly) innate sense of time, and we often have to manually construct the "natural" narrative of sequenced events from its raw component parts. In doing so we must face a lower-level reality: that the West's "civilized" conception of time—which we ordinarily think of as a purely physical property of the world around us—is in fact almost entirely metaphorical.

Cognitive linguist George Lakoff at the University of California at Berkeley discusses such metaphors in his widely read article "The Contemporary Theory of Metaphor."* For example, the following statements (in italics) from Lakoff's article accurately describe pieces of our common conception of time,

---

*George Lakoff, "The Contemporary Theory of Metaphor," in *Metaphor and Thought*, edited by Andrew Ortony (Cambridge, UK: Cambridge University Press, 1993), 202–51.

but have little to do with the actual physics of atomic motion that underlie the reality of time:

"Times are things [in the physical world]." Okay, sure. But if 2:35 P.M. is a physical thing, how much does it weigh? Where is it? *"The passing of time is motion." "Future times are in front of the observer; past times are behind the observer."* Yes, but what does time *actually* have to do with being in front of us or behind us, or passing us by? (Hint: absolutely nothing, except if, for example, we are walking, and time is motion.) Our physical future might just as easily lie behind us to the east, or over our heads in the penthouse apartment above us. And doesn't time also pass for a rock sitting in the desert? *"He stayed there [e.g., in that stage of his life] a long time."* Where, exactly, on Earth is he staying?

For a concussive who is struggling to understand something as simple as a friend saying, *"I'll see you next Tuesday at 4:30,"* the ubiquitously metaphorical conceptions of time are both suspect and elusive. In my case I would experience rapid thought processes such as: *Time is like motion. So it's like a train passing. And if I'm standing on the platform, then 4:30 Tuesday is like where the train is headed to down the tracks—so there will be some billboard there as the train later passes it, and that is my future.* And then, of course, I would struggle to visualize how some place I was supposed to be, such as my friend's house next to the train tracks, relates to the square in a calendar with a number (day of the month) in it, and what the symbol *4:30* (four-colon-thirty) has to do with it.

While all this thinking was going on under the hood, like Leonard in the movie I would smile and nod and say, *"Sure, 4:30 on Tuesday,"* knowing all the while that I had no idea what the phrase meant, that the effort to understand it was interfering with my balance, and that I was hoping to figure out how to get it into my simple calendar so I could better "deal with it later" before the nausea from the internal visualizing of the moving objects (such as the train) got too great to bear. And, of course, if my friend were to start saying something else, I might have a moment of internal desperation trying to process the *"4:30 Tuesday"* soon enough that I didn't lose either the *"4:30 Tuesday"* or whatever the new spoken input was.

For most of us, time is stored as a partially ordered collection of vignettes with a much stronger sense of before-and-after ordering than there is any sense of an immutable "continuous ether" in which these scenes are parked. To make sense of the narrative sequence, then, most of us will visualize not only the individual scenes themselves, but also a visual/spatial representation of them across a metaphorical "time" spectrum—from the earliest scene, through the present, and into the future. We can illustrate this by having you "point to" three scenes representing (1) when you got up this morning, (2) the present moment, and (3) tonight when you will go to bed. The chances are that you have some symbolic, highly *spatial* way of keeping these three scenes ordered (at least partially) according to time. You may have some kind of left-to-right ordering, a high-to-low ordering, or a foreground-to-background distinction. Or, you may have something much more abstract. The point is that you have *some* symbolic way to place such scenes in sequence. Ordinarily these will be located in three different areas in the physical space around you.

Because of the visual nature of these representations, shifting through the indexes of all these ordered scenes that make up the flow of time may greatly tax the already overworked visual/spatial processing systems in a concussive's brain. And as we are seeing in so many different ways, for concussives this visual processing is often *the* scarce resource that has to be jealously hoarded if they are to even minimally get through the day. Those dealing with concussives may, for this reason, find even the most naturally organized among them reluctant to make plans, to set dates, and to engage in activities such as scheduling their days.

An additional problem that I myself had, and that other concussives may share, was that under brain stress I lost the basic concept of before and after—of *ordering*—because I lost about half of what numbers meant. The *cardinality* of a set of items (in this case, time-stamped events)—the quantity of them, a more basic concept—was still intact, but the *ordinality* of them—the ordering of them—was gone. These two concepts are quite elemental in our thinking. If we consider the number "five," for example, it has both properties inherent in it: On the one hand it represents, say, the five children I have, the quantity of them, the set of five. On the other hand, it also represents the "fifth-ness" of my fifth child—*after* the fourth child—and thus implies an ordering. This loss of one's natural ability to order events can be quite troubling when it comes to making sense of narrative and the metaphors of time.

Imagine again the three scenes representing when you got up this morning, the current moment, and when you will go to bed tonight. The morning and evening scenes are very distinctly *not now*, and as such they live only as intellectual fabrications in your imagination. Compared with what is before your eyes and ears in this present moment, you can see that the *this-morning* and *this-evening* scenes are quite symbolic in nature—scenes filled with iconic representations of those parts of the real scene that are important: bed covers, sunlight or darkness, toothbrushes, clothes, what the floor looks like, and so on. It is also possible that, unlike the present moment, you have the perspective of looking *at* yourself—observing yourself in the narrative scene—rather than through the perspective of looking out *from* your own eyes. If so, this is de facto proof of the iconic nature of the images.

But now imagine yourself as a concussive who has lost the ability to "see" these elaborate spatial relationships. Now, instead of a natural, innately ordered progression of events, time becomes a *right-now* chaotic jumble of randomly inter-mixed scenes. Most troubling is the mixing up of those future scenes, which have been imagined—for the purpose of setting goals and creating plans—and those past scenes, which have already occurred, and are being stored as data. (Though note, very specifically not in a delusional way—the problem is sequencing, not knowing what is real.)

Lastly, an additional difficulty for a concussive may be in recognizing that a formerly future scene has now arrived. Consider that for most people, if their spouse has told them to be sure and mail a letter today, they'll form a picture of mailing the letter. Their body will, sooner or later, be prompted by the letter-mailing daemon that has been hovering around since morning waiting to match reality with that future image they have formed. To wit: when they enter the kitchen later in the day, the scene *reminds* them of the letter-mailing goal, they will open the kitchen drawer, take out the letter, and go outside to put it in the mailbox for pickup.

For a concussive, if the gestalt meaning, and context, of the current scene in the kitchen is missing because of visual system brain fatigue, the letter-mailing daemon may still sense some kind of match and try to break through to the drawer-opening mechanism, but ultimately can't. But the concussive is meanwhile growing unsettled, because she knows there is something wrong. This processing breakdown requires additional resources to sort out, in a downward spiral, and the visual processing now also deteriorates as visual-symbolic resources are used up trying to make sense of the kitchen, the unsettled feeling, and the repeated attempts to retrieve "something" that just isn't there. The balance system now gets affected, for the reasons we've discussed above, and nausea may set in because of it.

In trying to figure out what to do, everything becomes *right now* for the concussive. Instead of triggering *What was it I should be remembering?*, processing might become *Here are my hands in front of me; here is the floor; the ceiling is above the floor; it is late morning; there is light coming in the window,* and so on, all the while knowing all this is important (the prompting from the letter-mailing daemon), but not knowing why.

Sooner or later a concussive will sort it out, and probably get the letter mailed, but let us make no mistake: asking a concussive to do something as simple as mailing a letter may be an especially draining way for them to start their day.

It was, of course, Nolan's dissection of the structure of time that was so difficult for me to witness in *Memento,* and which caused me to identify so strongly with the experience of the main character: Leonard and I shared a sense of the literal, *right-now* nature of time, with all other temporal relationships being more or less a mystery that required intense intellectual effort to disentangle—a fictional portrayal that was yet truly evocative of my real-life experience.

CALENDARS AND THE INABILITY TO PLAN. Prior to the crash I was a skilled internal planner. Despite an appearance of chaos in my life—caused by my tendency to take on many big projects at the same time—I had a strong sense of how long those projects would take, and how they should best be interleaved both with one another, and with the many short-term goals I was also pursuing. I was the ultimate multitasker.

Within days of the crash, this intuitive planning skill disappeared completely. The way it disappeared, and my particular—and extreme—struggles with planning after the accident, are revealing. We can best understand my difficulties by first looking at four aspects of time, and also the way time relates to calendars: concepts that we typically take for granted, and which are crucial for planning.

First, as discussed, we tend to think of time as being linear: there was a yesterday, there is a now, there is a future. An important extension of this idea, crucial to developing plans, is the concept of *causality*, which comes with the constraint that earlier events can *cause* later events, but never the reverse.* Because I could no longer see the relationship between events, I was also generally unable to form images of causality, and of causal chains.

Second, in the modern world we associate geometry with blocks of sequenced time. Rectangles on a page—the days of a

---

*Though for scientific readers with an open mind, I can refer to studies of time-reversed causality that at least suggest this may not be the last word on cause and effect: D. I. Radin, (2011), "Predicting the Unpredictable: 75 Years of Experimental Evidence," in D. Sheehan (Ed)., *Frontiers of Time: Quantum Retrocausation* (American Institutes of Physics, forthcoming), and Daryl J. Bem, "Feeling the Future: Experimental Evidence for Anomalous Retroactive Influences on Cognition and Affect," *Journal of Personality and Social Psychology* 100(3) (March 2011): 407–25 (though not yet replicated). Thus modern science raises additional questions about why concussives—who operate closer to unfiltered reality—may have trouble with time.

calendar—are associated with, for example, the rising and set-ting of the sun each day. But this is a complex relationship: the unseeable spinning motion of the earth; the interplay of shad-ows and light and dark; the memory that tells us this day is *like* one that came before, and the logic that predicts it is *like* the one that will come tomorrow. And the calendar-geometry gets more complex: the artificial grouping of a line of days into rectangular seven-day weeks, rectangular weeks into square months, and layered 2D square months into a depth of 3D years, each represented on the page symbolically. As a concus-sive, when my brain was fatigued, I couldn't "see" the shapes in a calendar, nor could I conceptualize their link to events in the natural world. How do you draw a line from a one-inch square to an eight-thousand-mile diameter spinning rock traveling around the distant sun? The representation held no meaning for me.

Third, we assume time sequences are universal. To wit: when it is four o'clock in the afternoon in the living room in my house, it is also four o'clock in my office at the university, and if it takes an hour to drive from my house to the univer-sity, it will be five o'clock when I get there. But when I am at home in my living room, it is not ordinarily possible to see, or feel, or otherwise physically sense my office. The idea that time unfolds identically as a sequence of parallel events in all locations at once is purely conceptual, having no experiential correlation in our here-and-now perception of the world. (That is, we are *here*, or *there*, but never both at the same time, so we must trust our imagined construct of what is happening, in parallel, in the other location.)

And yet I came to understand that it is possible to be intel-ligent, and logical, and cogent, without having a concept of the universal nature of time, because when my brain grew fatigued I would lose it. Instead I would move down one level to a series of disconnected images: of time moving through the vehicle of a set of ordered images both at home, and differentially at the office, but without any intuitive sense that the events unfolding in each location were linked. To create time—to make it useful for planning where I needed to be, and when—I had to link the paired series of images together manually, consciously, using reasoning, and logic, and the memory that at one time I knew how it all fit together.

Lastly, we use numbers to represent both quantities and sequences of time, and while these concepts are intertwined, they are not the same. For example, when we make an appointment to have a suit of wedding clothes tailored on the eighth, we will want to schedule this appointment *before* our wedding on the fifteenth, and we care primarily about the before-and-after ordering of the dates—not the fact that 15 minus 8 yields an intervening period of 7 days. But when we schedule a week's vacation in California, we *are* primarily concerned that the start day and end day are seven days apart.

After the crash I lost almost all reliable representation of the above concepts—especially the linking of the natural world to geometric shapes and numbers on a page, making the use of a normal calendar impossible.

And yet I always had some *memory of having known* what a calendar was, and how to use it. So, in this way I was able to fake conversations about days, and weeks, and times, and even, in some cases, to successfully make an appointment without any real conceptual understanding of what I was doing. (As an analogy, consider that Google software is able to accurately translate the sentence "The dog is hungry" into German, but it has no more meaning to the software than does the sentence "Sewing is blue.")

In my daily life I had to very much stick to routines: For example, I would meet with a counselor, Dr. Miller, at 9:00 *every other Wednesday* for practical advice on how to manage life with brain damage. If I more-or-less figured that it was the right week, then I would go to see him. If it turned out to be the wrong Wednesday, then I would sit in his waiting room, he would not be there, and I would go home. This worked: I wasted quite a few mornings driving to a nonexistent appointment, but I almost never missed the appointments that I did have.

But if Dr. Miller had to change the appointment to another day—say Thursday at 10:00—this was very difficult for me. I might, for example, find myself staring at a card in my hand that said, "Next appointment, Thursday, February 8th, 10:00 A.M.," and I would be on the phone saying into his voicemail: "I see that I have an appointment on Thursday, February eighth, at ten A.M. I believe then that I am not coming on Wednesday, but I am not quite sure what that means. So, if this is not correct, please call me." Then I would call back days later, again holding the card, and say, "Today is Thursday. It is nine o'clock. I will be coming to your office to arrive at ten o'clock. I have a card here that says I am supposed to come to your office at ten o'clock, but I am not sure what that means. If I should not be driving to your office now, please call me back."

Then I would arrive at his office at ten o'clock, holding the card in my hand that said this was the time for me to be at his office, and I still was not confident that I was in the right place at the right time. Ten o'clock meant very little to me.

Thursday meant very little to me. The relationship between figures and dates written on a card, and my wristwatch (which gave both the date and time), meant little to me. The relationship between my wristwatch and the real world meant little to me.

It was not until two years after the crash, after a concerted, intense, and debilitating monthlong effort, that I was able to come up with something I thought might work: a simple, printed, one-page-per-month calendar where I numbered the days myself by hand. With difficulty, I gradually taught myself to use it . . . sort of. But until my recovery years later, my rudimentary use of the calendar was almost purely through procedural pattern matching, and with no linking to the underlying concepts and metaphors we use to manipulate time in the modern world.

I believe that many concussives have similar difficulties with calendars, dates, planning, and the conceptual building blocks of time. For example, the famous linebacker Junior Seau was believed to have exhibited signs of brain injury after his retirement, prior to his suicide. In a *San Diego Union-Tribune* article that ran in late 2012, Seau's family talked about how hard it was to schedule anything on the calendar with him. His wife is reported as saying, "His keeping appointments had gotten progressively worse. The kids and I would call him three, four, or five times a day to remind him about their games or events. We'd say, 'Don't forget about tonight.' He'd say, 'Where is it?' And we'd say, 'We've told you 50 times. Go back into your text messages and look.' It got to the point where you couldn't tell him the day before an event and expect him to remember."

THE BUILDING BLOCKS OF COGNITION AND THE METACOGNITIVE VOICE

COGNITIVE SLOWING. One of the recurring difficulties that would arise after the crash was *cognitive slowing*, as though my brain's mainspring were simply winding down. I would increasingly experience both cognition, and the movement of my body, in super slow motion. My brother Will recently commented on noticing this when he visited about a year after the crash:

> I remember us sitting in a restaurant and I watched you reach for the salt shaker. You were concentrating intensely. First you looked at the salt shaker, then your hand, then the salt shaker again. As you slowly guided your hand across the table in this way, it was as though you were inventing—for the first time and from first principles—the whole idea of space, and movement

through that space to pick up an object. Really striking. Really weird.

This slow-motion effect could be extreme. During one test at a rehabilitation center several years after the crash, a specialist attempted to measure my reaction time, as I responded to visual displays on a computer screen by pressing keys on the keyboard. Despite our best efforts I was ultimately deemed untestable: under the visual/spatial demands of the test my reaction times to press a key would go from less than a second, to several seconds, to a minute, to five minutes. At that point the software would time out, assuming we had abandoned the test. Internally I was still going through the same procedures as I did for the one-second response—but it was now taking me three hundred times as long to manage the steps of moving my hand.

This kind of general cognitive slowing often resulted when I had to push myself through difficult balance problems. For example, after being forced to take a commuter train home in 2004 it took me four hours to come down the stairs from the train platform, and walk the one mile home from there. I noted my progress by following individual leaves along the hedges, and individual bricks on the buildings next to the sidewalk as I walked home.

This slowing was at the same time attended by a real-time ability to observe and record my experience through what Donalee Markus, Ph.D. (whom we will meet later), calls the *meta-cognitive voice*. This voice is very much part of what makes us human: it is the continual voice-over that offers commentary on our place in the world, allows us to be sympathetic to the experiences of others, and gives us the very human capability of self-reflection.

For example, as you are reading this passage, your meta-cognitive voice allows you to simultaneously *observe that you are sitting here reading.*

The metacognitive voice also allows us to change our narrative perspective: you can imagine yourself sitting at your kitchen table eating breakfast, with your hands and plate in front of you. Then, with a slight internal flick of a switch, you can again observe yourself sitting at the same table eating, only now from across the room.

We now find a unique juxtaposition of circumstances: On the one hand, my cognition slowed enough that I could reflect on individual processing steps that might ordinarily take place at subsecond speeds—well below the threshold of being able to discriminate them. On the other hand, my *recording* of these steps took place at the full speed of a strong intellect. Thus I had the rare opportunity to watch the unfolding of raw and stunningly complex human cognition in slow motion, and yet at the same time record it in normal speed as a trained observer who has knowledge of computational systems.

THE METACOGNITIVE OBSERVER. Before we look at some of these extreme details of cognition I witnessed, there are two additional factors about me, and my individual brain makeup, that might be an important part of the record. For these we have to make a slight digression.

First, when I was a child my IQ was reportedly extremely high; I finished all of my district's high school math curriculum on my own, sitting out in the hall in the sixth grade as an eleven-year-old, and then began riding my bike up to the University of California at Berkeley to sit in on math and physics classes. Although I never made much use of these talents—spending the first part of my life as a musician—I was always a natural at manipulating symbols, especially in geometric ways.

Second, I had a sort of transcendent experience when I was fourteen years old that may give clues to my ability to record my slow-motion concussion experiences:

After spending an afternoon lying on the fringes of a golf course with my friend Cathy, watching beautiful white cumulus clouds roll past, and near what later turned out to be thought of by some as a "spiritual focal point" in the Berkeley Hills, I had an odd sensation of splitting in two. The "me" that we typically think of, the locus of consciousness—perhaps a form of the metacognitive voice—was freed up to "stay in the clouds," so to speak, and to observe the tiniest details of the experience of life unfolding. At the same time, the "me" part of my mind that intentionally got through the day—corresponding to the part of ourselves that thinks, and holds conversations, and goes to school, and sleeps—went about its business exactly as usual.

This was very much like what happens when we drive a car down the highway—it's not necessary for us attend to the details of the road, freeing us up to hold conversations with passengers or perhaps pay attention to what's on the radio. In this case my whole life, and me getting through it, was on autopilot, while the conscious me, the *real* me, was able to simply observe the true beauty of the whole system—with me in it—unfolding. I tried to explain my circumstances to others, but no one was much interested. None of them noticed anything different or "dreamy" about me. I completed my homework assignments in the usual way. I participated in classes at school. I had normal conversations with my family members. I thought up jokes and goofed around with my friends in the usual way. I was in all ways entirely *present*. Yet at the same time the *real* me was simply watching all of this go on, attending not only to the temporal me working through my life, but also to the most minute details of the interplay of light on leaves, of the choreography of motion in the world around me, the many scents that we almost universally ignore, the sound and smell and essential grace of people with whom I was interacting, and so on. I watched myself fall asleep at night, and I watched myself wake up in the morning.

I felt as though I had chanced on some kind of enlightenment. This marvelous experience lasted for three days, and then gradually went away over the next two. I longed to recapture this dual nature, and tried for many years, but it only returned once, three years later, and then only for a day.

It's not important to determine whether this was a minor mystical gift to an impressionable young man, or a small perturbation in the posterior parietal cortex (the part of the brain to which neuroscience sometimes attributes such experiences). The point is that one way or another this youthful adventure in transcendent metacognition was de facto proof that we really are capable of observing ourselves in great detail without necessarily interfering with what we ordinarily think of as consciousness. It might also suggest some oddity in my own brain that later allowed me to take the detailed notes that are the basis of this book, even while suffering from sometimes quite striking concussion symptoms.

WHO ARE MY CHILDREN? THE ANALOGICAL BRAIN. Let's fast-forward now to the fall of 2007—eight years after the crash. Largely because of an inability to filter out the continual chatter of my highly verbal three-year-old—who was almost exclusively in my care by this time—I was nearing the end. To maintain my life as a full-time professor and full-time single parent, I needed to be very crafty about using what few cognitive resources I had left with maximum efficiency. So I devised an assessment test that I gave to myself every morning before heading off to work. I would sit in the living room and ask myself, "What are the names of my children?" On normal brain days, I could list the names of my five children in six seconds, and I knew that I could take on some challenges that day. On bad brain days it would take me more than three minutes, and even then I was not quite certain of the answer. On those days I knew to avoid any kinds of demands other than those of being a father, and teaching my classes.

Even on bad days, I was completely *logical*. I knew exactly what was going on. I was simply experiencing the physical breakdown of my brain resulting in an extreme slowing of cognition. And yet, at the same time, as noted above, *I could observe the process in the normal way.*

What follows are selections from a much longer composite record based on a number of different days; every one of the mental processes otherwise took place exactly as given here. This record gives us a window into both the building blocks of cognition and the stunning analogical processing capabilities of the human brain that I believe go on under the hood at blazing speed, without our noticing, twenty-four hours a day. It also lays the groundwork for understanding how Donalee Markus's analogical mental puzzles (which we'll see later) can help a plastic brain to recover from traumatic injury—even after eight years.

Two themes developed. First, it is my strong intuition that for the most part, the *substance* of my train of thought was following normal cognitive patterns, albeit in extreme slow motion. It is true that there were occasional cognitive-symbolic deficits from the TBI that required alternate problem-solving paths: occasionally I would search for an answer, or try to re-trieve a concept, and nothing would come to mind, so I would have to try something else. But I believe these to be the excep-tion, and not the rule.

Second, when working on the problem, and developing par-tial results that had to be saved for later, I had the most tangible feeling of a limited "working memory" space, which would auto-matically empty itself to make room for new thinking results.* Thus, if I didn't want to lose the bigger picture surrounding my current train of thought, I would have to regularly leave off my ongoing computations, go back to the beginning, and refresh all of my intermediate results and problem-solving paths. In the ex-ample below I would have to refresh every eight to thirty sec-onds. As the speed of my processing increased, so did the frequency and speed of my refreshes. On six-second days, when my impairment was at a minimum, I had the sense that I would refresh just as many times as in the example below, but so rapidly that I couldn't perceive it. For the sake of brevity I'll only give the details of the first refresh below, then leave out the other (ul-timately eighteen) refreshes that occurred during the following composite episode.

This passage contains only a fifth of the notes I have extant for what would amount to a full, single event. In the unabridged passage from which this excerpt is drawn—in what I strongly believe to be a relatively normal path to determining who my children are—I introduce several hundred concepts, make

---

*There are many extremely detailed measures of working memory in cognitive psychol-ogy. I use the term loosely here to refer to my explicit experience, but offer no commen-tary about any formal, testable properties in this context.

analogical jumps among many of them, generate images for most of the concepts, and backtrack numerous times—abandoning those particular paths as fruitless. As mentioned, on a normal day, this will have taken six seconds—much too fast for us to observe; on a bad brain day, such as in the exposition below, more than three minutes. It is this latter that gives us our unique window into how the analogical brain works. We might wonder how we can "ordinarily" fit such a staggering number of reasoning steps into six seconds, but this is understandable if we consider that humans are well capable of *perceiving* information at a minimum of something like twenty-four frames a second. (Below this *critical flicker fusion threshold*, for example, we begin to have problems with flicker detection in video streams.) Neural signals can propagate through brain networks in thousandths of a second.*

Here, then, is an excerpted, composite record of my sample brain-assessment test:

> I come downstairs in the early morning and sit in front of the coffee table in my living room. I start the timer on my wristwatch and ask the question,
>
> "What are the names of my children?"
>
> *Blank.* Nothing comes to mind. I simply *hear* the sound of the question. I wait for a while, but then instead of an answer I get a different question, represented visually in front of my eyes, black font on a white rectangular background:
>
> "Do I have children?"

---

*In fact, our perception rate is *far* higher in many instances: in working out the debate between analogue and digital music recordings, for example, it has become clear that we hear changes in sound quality that occur in ten thousandths of a second, and perhaps even *far* less than that.

There is no answer to this question either. But this is related, and simpler, because it is . . . *binary—yes or no.* I see the word "Binary," also black on a white background. But I am cloudy on what it means. I try to recall the geometric *shape* of a binary question. It takes me a while, but finally I see what a binary question is, the shape of it: upper right—*yes,* stretching diagonally to the lower left—*no,* and the whole image sitting just to the upper left of my internal center visual field. Because I can *see binary,* I can now also *feel binary.*

O.K., I think to myself, I've got: *binary question.*

I am not sure of the answer to this new question, but it seems that if I do not have children it will become obvious anyway, so there is no sense in choosing that I do not. Thus I can *assume* that I have children, and if this is not right then something else will take care of that other path. But I am cloudy on exactly what the other path is and what will take care of it.

I now must grasp enough of the concept of *assumption* to allow me to continue. This takes a while. Then . . .

Got (sort of): *assumption.*

I can feel a daemon being created to attend to what happens if the assumption turns out to be false, but I resist it: I don't want to waste precious resources in case the assumption turns out to be true.

So now, assuming that I *do* have children, how does one go about figuring out who they are?

No answer. So I have to think about it.

It seems that a typical way would be to figure out *how many*. If I can recall how many children I have, then I know I have them.

What would an answer to "how many?" look like? *Not sure.* I have to think about this. I wait.

Then: *A number.* If I can answer how many, it will be a number.

No number comes to mind, and while I am waiting for one, I feel the pressure to recall the context of my thinking, so that I don't lose my place. So . . .

[Refresh number one] I place a marker where I am, and go back to the beginning of the problem to recut the routes so that I can recall what I am trying to answer. Refresh: *Who are my children?* Refresh: *Do I have children?* Refresh: *Binary question.* Refresh: *Assumption.* Refresh: *Stop the false-assumption daemon.* Refresh: *How many children?* Refresh: *Answer will be a number.* Refresh: *No number is coming to mind.*

Now, back to the current problem. Something about *numbers* is important. I need some numbers, and I need to retrieve something about how numbers work.

Numbers have *order.* I'm not sure what order is (or sequence), but I know that numbers have it. I get that numbers have cardinality—naming a quantity—and this seems loosely related to numeracy, but what is ordinality?

Nothing comes to mind.

[Refresh number two (hereafter, etc.)]

[Skipping ahead . . .]

I have formed a vague idea of what *order* is: something about *bigger and smaller.* But while (a) I do not remember what bigger and smaller are, or what they have to do with one another, and (b) I do not recall what bigger and smaller have to do with numbers, or order, I *do* know that (c) there are answers to these questions, that (d) the answers are important, and that (e) I have known these answers before. I work on this for a while.

[Skipping far ahead . . .]

Even though, to save resources, I have managed to suppress starting an "Assumption Daemon" to know what to do if my assumption (that I do have children, as opposed to the binary opposite option that I don't) turns out to be false, a different daemon springs to life: one that *worries that I have not started such an Assumption Daemon.* This annoying "Worry Daemon" gets more insistent, popping into my consciousness from time to time, until I finally give in and formulate the clear thought: *assumption* means that I might be wrong; this whole exercise might be for nothing; I've assumed that I have children; if I don't have children, then I cannot name them, and I am done. The *Worry Daemon* now goes away. It is replaced by the *Assumption Daemon* I was trying to avoid triggering, which lingers around looking for an instance of me realizing that I don't have children, in which case it will leap into consciousness to remind me that this whole line of reasoning is invalid.

[Skipping ahead . . .]

I'm still struggling with *order*. Because it is such a low-level, elemental concept, it is hard for me to reconstruct. I am on the verge of getting it though, and am unwilling to risk losing everything by going to refresh. So I postpone the refresh. Instead, I fire off a "Refresh Reminder Daemon" so I can, literally, "deal with that later." Then I immediately get back to the problem at hand.

As I continue to work, the *Refresh Reminder Daemon* continually makes me anxious in an undifferentiated way (I can feel this anxiety in the muscles of my upper back, and in my breathing), and periodically it also intrudes into consciousness to say, "Refresh! We HAVE to refresh!"

[Skipping ahead . . .]

I've finally made progress: from *order*, to *numbers*, to *ordinality* [if objects can be represented by numbers, they can be ordered], to *precedence* [a number can be greater, or "more important," than another number based on its qualities of *numberness*], to *relationship* [between two adjacent numbers], to *sequence* [a collection of relationships], to list [the instantiation of a sequence by actual objects]. I form the substantial concept that if I can make an *ordered list* of symbolic placeholders, then replace the placeholders with my children, I'll know who they are.

This is a *chunking* point—where a master concept replaces all its constituent smaller ones: having gotten to *ordered list*, and the concept of filling it in with my children, I no longer need to keep track of *order, numbers, ordinality, precedence, relationship,* and *sequence.* The *Refresh Reminder Daemon* now seizes its chance. I've reached a breathing point. I clear out the unneeded intermediate concepts and refresh the remaining context. The daemon, having completed its mission, dies off. [That is, I now go back to normal periodic refreshes.]

Over the next ninety seconds I cover a lot of ground. In trying to instantiate the ordered list with my children, I begin to associate the numbers that will [far in the future] be associated with their ages. I see these numbers as black symbols floating around over a white background, but I have a problem getting them to settle into an order: because of my concussion-induced *hemispatial neglect* I have once again lost the right-hand side of my world. Thus I am trying to create a list with a left side, but no right side. I realize this can't work, and in a marvel of plastic cognitive adaptability automatically begin my search for an alternate representation. The question arises: *how do I represent a left-to-right sequence/list when there is no right-hand side to my world?*

In an episode of synesthesia I start replacing numbers with sounds, and then mix the sounds with colors. In the context of *sound-color* I am able to revisit the idea of a *sequence* now as a sequence of colors: cool colors on the left blending toward hot colors on the right (like the sequence in a color wheel). This frees me from the *left-is-less* and *right-is-more* number-line rule. I don't understand quite what *smaller* and *bigger* are, but I nonetheless manage to tease out that *smaller on the left* and *bigger on the right* is part of my problem. Ultimately, after numerous steps I come up with the following: I use *weightiness* on the left (because my left side is substantial) and *ephemeralness* on the right (because my right-hand side is cloudy, fuzzy) as the relationship between elements of my list. I am using sound-color, like musical sequences from low to high, and like having the big bass strings of a piano on the left, and the smaller high-pitched strings on the right, to form my ordered list of elements. I know that I have *reversed* my number-ordered list so that smaller is now on the right. I don't really know what *reversed* means, and have to work this out after the fact, keeping this parallel representation—*reversed*—active the whole time I am using the list. Gradually, the music/sound/color representation recedes (though it was essential in creating the initial reversed list), and I solidify the concept of a *reversed number list*. I still can't see the right side of my world, including the right side of the list, but I've been clever in using this to mean "less on the right."

After another long sequence I now wrestle with the concept of *two* lists: a symbolic one in my head, a *real* one in the outside world, and the relational linking of the two together. I struggle with the concept of mapping analogue symbols for items in the real world—my children—into the empty list I've created in my head. *Inside* I am creating, dreaming, making things up; *outside* I am seeing, recalling, perceiving. I move my visual/spatial representation back and forth between the two, and as I do so, my eyes actually move, and refocus, following my thoughts.

This difference in perspective between two such lists is significant. You can see it with the following exercise: Imagine, in your head, a word list—the names of places you have lived; now imagine those same places on the grid of the earth and mentally point in the direction of each of them as you work through the list. These are two entirely different representations. The first is purely symbolic, but the second is a real-world corollary of the first, with spatial sense, and direction, and geometric relationships between each of the cities and your current location on Earth. And once we have established the two lists, we can link them together: the city-name words in the internal list each to a real city on the face of the earth in the external list.

This linking between the real, physical world and our internal, symbolic representation of it is something that we ordinarily manage with intuitive grace. We move elegantly along the mappings from one to the other, and switch with ease between the quite different representations. But here we see that I've lost that ability. Instead, I must explicitly define the relationship between the two.

At this point we come to an interesting revelation, and I want to call special attention to it. I had, by this time in my life, come to believe that I had no hope of ever recovering from the brain damage. Instead, I focused on trying to improve my effectiveness by being clever with the limited brain resources I retained. As part of my efforts, I had decided it was important to recognize when to *give up*. This was an entirely foreign concept to me, but under the circumstances was appropriate, and necessary. The mantra went something like, *You have brain damage, Clark. There are things that you simply can no longer manage, so don't try to. Don't push yourself too far!* I had practiced "giving up" for several years now—letting go of some of my responsibility—but it was contrary to my nature and never came naturally. At this point in the exercise, the intensity of my mental work is grinding my tired brain down, and I start to experience head pain and nausea. I'm perspiring from the effort. Several times I am reminded of the rule:

Clark, you are in pain, so now YOU MUST STOP.

This is annoying. I know intuitively that it will take up precious resources to figure out what *stopping* means, and how to integrate *stopping* with reaching my goal. I don't have time for that. But as I continue, and my distress level rises, my need to address the rule becomes overwhelming. I finally pause to briefly mull this over.

But now something really interesting happens: in considering "Should I stop now?" another absolutely clear, elemental rule pops up:

Clark NEVER GIVES UP.

So who am I? I ask myself.

I can't get it. *I have two conflicting rules.* It's too much work to figure out, and is draining too much energy from the problem at hand. In the end I stop trying to be someone I don't understand, and just continue instead with solving the problem. The increasing pain, and the well-intentioned new rules, are nothing next to *who I am.*

But what are the implications here? This core identity—the guy who just never gives up—is integrated into my being at the lowest level of cognition—the same level at which the concepts of *left and right* and *inside and outside* are stored. This is not part of some narrative personal story, nor is it some high-level learned trait. It is a most basic, elemental, *cognitive* part of me.*

Over the next sixty seconds I work through—among other concepts—the idea that I have a *set* of children that will be mapped one-to-one into the slots in my internal list; that sets have cardinality (the countable number of items in the set); that children have ages; and so on. I get stymied waiting for a number to rise up out of the ether that will set an upper limit on the *range* of elements in my list. I get tied up with the idea of a *zero-length list*, and the *Assumption Daemon* leaps out to claim this as an instance of the failed assumption that I have children.

At one point I simply wait, perched, doing nothing at all except letting the mysterious cauldron of my brain boil away. After a while, and after I've clearly formed my question, some hidden process takes place, and the number "5" floats up out of the ether: I have five children. There is no association to be made. The process is atomic: one moment there is nothing, the next moment the visual image of the number "5" is floating across my internal field of vision.

I don't fully know what "5" means, but five is like the five fingers on my left hand, facing me. Fingertips, like ovals, like faces, people, the history of primitive people, tribes, families, parents, children, oldest children, *first* children, biggest, oldest on the left. Reversed list. Oldest child, oval face, flesh-colored, like the thumb on my left hand facing me. I see the face of my oldest daughter, superimposed. I can't access her name, but I do *know* that I know her name.

---

*We might ask: how do we address it when someone has, instead, an elemental concept of himself as the one who "can't do it"? If my experience is anything to go on, we'd have to look at the deepest levels of symbolic cognition to make changes to such a built-in program. We're talking about shapes and colors and primitive relationships here—not the story of one's family life.

I've gone back to refresh sixteen times at this point.

I release many items, partial results that I have stored in working memory. The *Assumption Daemon* dies off, because having seen one child, I know that I have children: I no longer have to consider taking an alternate path that would have been necessary had my assumption turned out to be false. I release the marker that I am still unclear about what *binary* means (yes/no—do I have children?). I let go of the ordinality and cardinality properties of numbers, because I need only the one number: five. My refresh list gets much shorter. I feel tangibly energized as my cognitive resources are freed up.

I retrieve the concept of male children (boys) and female children (girls). I bind my daughter, Nell, to my left thumb, palm facing me, which is hard because this is backward—the *reversed list*, with the *oldest* (biggest) on the *left*. I have to physically "look" her into this binding by staring intently at my thumb. I speak her name:

"Um. My oldest child is Nell."

It has been two and a half minutes of intense concentration and I've just named my first child.

I get the sentence out, but the effort of translating thought into speech causes all of my visual memory of the problem I am working on to disappear. I have to go back and retrieve many of the markers again, and recut the channels. I get back the image of Nell, and then, over time, in sequence, the images of my other four children appear. There are two additional difficulties, one primarily linguistic and the other arithmetical: My boys are named *Peter* and *Paul*, they are often together—they are very close—and the alliteration of the "P" sound at the beginning of their names further binds them to each other. Because Peter is the second oldest, Lucy the third, and Paul the fourth, I have to slip Lucy in between the two boys. But she is a girl, and she has an "L" sound in her name, so I have to fight against the "P" symmetry, and the "boy" symmetry, to get her into the right place. In struggling with this problem I again lose Nell, and have to go back quite a ways to retrieve her. I have even more trouble with my youngest, Erin. It takes significant time to add her to the list. The children are aged *18, 16, 14, 12,* and Erin—*3*. She is not an even-numbered age. She acts differently from the rest because she is so much younger. There is a gap to get to her. Each of these factors upsets the symmetry of the structures I am building to hold my children—to hold the symbols of them in my mind's eye—so that I can name them.

My retrieval of the children as I fill in the list also involves partially seeing a visual montage of their life activities—which is part of who they are, like their names.

I say aloud, "My son, Peter."

As I do so the visual images of Peter, and Nell, fly off like startled birds. Translating the image of Peter into a physical utterance requires so much cognitive "horsepower" that I cannot maintain the imagery at the same time.

Finally I get to "Erin, age *3*."

I'm exhausted. I've named my five children—maybe. I can't see them all at once, and by the time I've named Erin, I can no longer really conceive of having named Nell. I am not able to speak their names and see their faces at the same time. I look at my watch: three and a half minutes. It's not a good day for taking on challenges.

The assessment test might take me anywhere from 6 to 210 seconds. Because the range of time covered such a spectrum, and because I went through the exercise so many times, I observed the process in many different ways. My strongest intuition is that, except for some of the deficits that coincidentally came with brain fatigue (e.g., the hemispatial neglect, and the synesthesia), *the process was the same* no matter how long it took, and that this record gives us a unique window into the massive low-level cognitive processing that goes on inside all of us throughout the day, beneath our consciousness—even for what appear to be simple mental tasks.

GETTING HOME / THE DOG THAT WASN'T. At times the juxtaposition of my internal and external lives was startling. An episode that occurred eight years after the crash illustrates how little my surface life—in which I was pursuing such normal activities as going to the movies—reflected the complex processing going on under the hood, which by this time was occasionally so bizarre as to be almost unreal.

At first glance, it might appear that I was finally losing touch with reality. In fact, on closer examination, the case can be made that while I was clearly impaired, I was actually operating *closer* to the true nature of raw, unfiltered "reality" than normals, doing my best to navigate our world without the powerful cognitive filters that do so much of the work for us by excluding most of our sensory input *before* it enters consciousness. Within this context, I was entirely lucid and logical.

The following episode illustrates more than a dozen distinct cognitive failures and workarounds, including some interesting *ideaesthesia* oddities (ideas mixing with senses), and difficulties mapping mental symbols to their real-world analogues, and then ends in a truly strange sequence that highlights an aspect of our inherent *linguistic* intelligence.

On this particular spring afternoon in 2007, Qianwei happened to be home between business trips—and she could stay with our daughter Erin. I took advantage of the rare opportunity and went to the movies to let the images roll past, with no requirement that I need make sense of them. My "deep batteries" were depleted from the grind of the long school year, and from being a virtual single parent. Going to the movies usually afforded me a little mental break, but for some reason this time the processing of dialogue and the visual input made things worse.

I left the theater's parking lot as the sun was setting, in the classic Toyota Supra cult-car I was considering restoring, to make the seven-minute, two-mile drive home. I had no trouble managing the car, but soon found that I did not recognize any of the visual landmarks around me. As had occasionally happened to me in the past, neither the streets nor the neighborhoods looked familiar, as though I were experiencing some kind of "building prosopagnosia"—face blindness for buildings. I could read the words on the street signs, but they too were simply empty patterns of letters. I could not figure out how to get home.

I thought that if I drove for a while I would start to recognize where I was. The problem was that I already *did* have a clear visual appraisal of my surroundings, and in one sense I knew *exactly* where I was—I just could not access that knowledge in any way that was useful. For example, I could have told you, "That's the YMCA where Paul plays basketball, and where my friend Liam saved a girl from drowning," but I could not *recognize* the Y or any other building, or place any of them in a larger visual context in a way that gave me a sense of having seen them before—I couldn't make a meaningful whole from the various pieces. And, the pieces were useless to me for navigation because without the "thingness" of them I didn't have any way to place them in the larger geography that made up my local world. When I read the names on the street signs, waiting for the meaning of the streets in the real world to come to me (their placement on the grid of the city, their usefulness in getting me home), nothing happened.

Very strange!

Over the course of the next hour I drove in slowly expanding circles around the downtown area. Finally, to at least get some NSEW grounding I drove (downhill) over to the shore of Lake Michigan, half a mile away, because I knew the lake formed the eastern boundary of the city, giving me a point of reference. Then, because of a 9:00 P.M. curfew along the lakeshore, I drove several blocks west and parked there on a side street. As I did so, I fired up a daemon charged with preserving my geometric orientation relative to the lake. Over the course of the succeeding hour, this *Orientation Daemon* slowly drained away at my remaining cognitive batteries. Roughly speaking, it was like an annoying voice in my head, interrupting every three or four seconds, quietly reminding me, *Lake Michigan is behind you, to the east, so you are now headed west. Don't forget!*

Using speed-dial six on my cell phone, I called Jake in San Diego to ask for help. He was in the middle of a challenging project at work, and impatient to get back to it.

"I don't get it," he said curtly. "You've never had trouble getting home before. Where are you?"

"I don't know, Jake," I said. "I don't recognize any of the streets or any of the buildings. I've driven in circles for an hour and am now facing west, away from the lake, which is several blocks behind me."

"Okay," he said, "we can work with that. Get out of the car. Walk to a street corner. Look around at what you see. Memorize the names on the street signs, then call me back."

It was ten minutes before I could initiate getting out of the car. Once out on the street, I had to hold on to the car, a parking-sign pole, and some hedges, to walk to the corner—seventy-five feet away. Visual, olfactory, auditory, and proprioceptive information was flooding in, but because my sensory filters were not working, I was getting everything all the time, and all at once, in one giant, flattened collection of small features from the environment. I couldn't form meaningful interpretations of what I was seeing. I was also having trouble extracting visual balance information from the environment, as twilight settled in, making it hard to walk.

So I did my best to simply keep all the objects I encountered in memory. After twenty minutes, exhausted, I got back to the car and reported the data to Jake. "I am next to a big house that has fourteen lights turned on in many rooms with no people, which I can see through the windows, so we know I am in a wealthy neighborhood. The curb has a circle and some orange letters spray-painted on it, probably from a previous street, gas, or water repair. There are tall hedges with thin branches and lots of small leaves."

Jake said, "Okay. Hedges. Paint. A big house by the lake. That doesn't help us much. Anything from the corner, where the street signs are?"

I told him, "I could make out what looked like an explosion of green leaves, and some white flowers. Putting them all together, I'm guessing it was a big bush, or a tree. Next to the tree there were signs on a pole."

"Okay. Good job," said Jake. "Were they street signs? Were there names?"

"I can't really say," I told him. "I am trying to tell you, but I can't. It is very difficult for me. Yes, there were two street signs. One of them was, well . . . it was . . . *Michigan*."

There were two immediate problems that had begun to plague me. The first was that the drain from the Lake Michigan Orientation Daemon (used to remember *east*) became significantly worse because I now had to disambiguate the internal visual symbol for *Lake Michigan* (i.e., starting with a capital *M*) from the nearly identical symbol for *Michigan Avenue*—the cross-street up at the corner to which I had just walked. Sorting out the cognitive interference between the two was wearing me down.

The second problem was even more disconcerting, and illustrates a form of *ideaesthesia* (not to be confused with the less accurate *synesthesia* in this case) that would sometimes crop up.* The street on which I was parked—corresponding to the other sign at the corner—was "Greenleaf." But I was having trouble discriminating the street name not only from the sight of the *green leaves* that were fluttering in the glow from the streetlight, but also from the *green spring scent* of the (green) leaves themselves and of the flowers, and even from the internal raw *shape* of *greenness* in my mind.

Nonetheless, with Jake's encouragement I might have been able to form the vocalization for "Greenleaf Street" if he had not, ironically, picked the one helping tactic that would put me over the edge. He asked, "Can you tell me what the color of the sign is, and what color the letters are? If you can describe the signs I'll at least know what city you're in."†

At this point a giant cognitive bell was lowered over my head and concussion-sprites began beating on it with hammers. Such cognitive pain from sensory and semantic flooding is difficult to describe, but it is quite real, and sometimes excruciating, nonetheless. Every part of my psyche wanted only to get away from it, but it is a spigot that cannot be turned off. I could not get away from Jake's question about the lettering on the sign—the answer to

---

*Imagine I gave you drawings of (1) a spiky figure, and (2) a gently curved line, and asked you to identify them as either a *Patiki-tiki* or a *Smoo*. Almost everyone would associate the spiky figure with the Patiki-tiki, and the curve with the Smoo, based on the *ideas* of spikiness and gentle curves. For me, at times of stress, such ideas, which affected perception and meaning, would blend with objects in the real world.
†Jake is expert in knowing things like what style and color of street sign each city uses.

which was: *white* letters on a *green* background. I couldn't escape the now echoing images of the green tree leaves blowing in the wind, or the scent of those leaves and their white flowers bleeding scent into the visual images, or the white letters forming the street name "Greenleaf," with its attendant aural image also bleeding into the sight and smell of the whole green and white chaotic jumble.

I struggled to keep from throwing up. I dropped the phone and put my hands over my ears to shut out all sound. I clamped my eyes closed as firmly as my face muscles would allow.

After a while, the hammer/bell pain subsided. I picked up the phone again. I very much wanted to answer Jake's question so he could get me home. I *knew* that I knew the answer to his question, but I also knew I was not going to be able to untangle the cognitive interference.

"I can't tell you about the signs," I said, "because of the tree."

"You mean the tree is covering the signs up?"

"No," I said, "I can see the signs fine, but I can't tell you what they say, or what color they are." (I meant, of course, that I literally could not *tell* Jake about the signs, even though I wanted to, and even though I knew the answers to his questions.)

"Okay," he said. "We aren't getting anywhere. Think about it, and call me back. I'll be here." Then he hung up.

Jake was clearly annoyed. He had asked me a straightforward question, to which I knew the answer, but which for my own baroque reasons I wasn't telling him. Understandably, a serious Guilt Daemon now started up, and began its own additional drain on the now dangerously diminished resources I was doing my best to conserve. This was a strong emotion, and repeatedly demanded a further slice of my brain's processing power every few seconds in an opportunistic way, competing with the other daemons still operating: *Did you correct your inexcusable and weird social action yet?*

Then two seconds later, *How about now? Did you finally decide to give Jake his answer?* Then, *Don't forget that Lake Michigan is behind you, to the east.* Then, *Lake Michigan is not the same as Michigan Avenue and you have to remember both . . .* , and so on.

So I shut everything down and sat in the car for a long time, staring at the Supra logo on my steering wheel and doing absolutely nothing.

Finally, sufficiently restored, I called Jake and told him that I was going to head west, away from the lake, and hope for the best. I stopped the car every few blocks and gave him an update. Eventually he pinpointed my location on Greenleaf Street, about a mile from my house.

An hour after leaving the lakeshore—more than two hours after leaving the theater—I finally made it back to the block where I lived. Jake stayed on the phone with me and guided me house by house down my street—a neighborhood I had known for twenty-five years but now seemed to be visiting for the first time. I had been so intent on getting home that I wasn't prepared for what followed: I didn't recognize my own house. There was no "home" at which to arrive. My heart started racing. Now what?

"Look, Jake," I said as I struggled out of the car, "this is really getting out of hand, and definitely scary. What if we've screwed up, and this is someone else's house? I need some kind of cover story in case I'm caught in the yard and some guy comes out wondering what I'm doing here."

Jake said, "Okay. *Just tell them that you are looking for your dog.*" The particular wording of his statement would later prove to be of seminal importance.

I walked up to the silent house, and verified the address with Jake. I struggled to get the key in the lock, but once in, it worked smoothly, and I was able to open the front door.

I sucked in my breath, and with the same feeling you would have breaking into someone else's house at night, I walked into the darkened living room. In a hushed voice I described the interior of the house to Jake, which included, rather distinctively, two pianos. Given the pianos, and the empirical fact that my key fit in the door, there was no doubt whatsoever—intellectually—that I was in my own house. But I felt none of the transformative and critically important *certainty* that would have been so effortlessly generated in a normal.

I went into the music room and sat down next to my record collection. I could easily have told you which pressings (indicated by the hand-etched lettering near the record label) of Rubinstein's *Carnaval* recording I had on the shelf, or described the sonic qualities of my original Reginald Kell Brahms Clarinet Quintet recording. My memory was fully intact. But without low-level apprehension of the visual/spatial *meaning* of my surroundings, I had no way to interact with them, no way to feel the place for them in my world. I didn't know what to do. I started to wonder where "my dog" was.

"It's like I've never been in this house before," I whispered over the phone. "I don't recognize anything, and I'm particularly worried that I don't see the dog." Jake had reached his limit. Satisfied that I was home, he understandably wanted to get back to work. *"Don't worry about the dog!"* he said impatiently before he hung up. Again, his choice of words proved to be important.

I sat for twenty minutes in the dark room, fretting. I was loath to go upstairs and see Qianwei and the kids, because of the nightmare scenario in which I would not recognize them either. After all, I already didn't recognize the house, plus I had no memory of our dog. Why couldn't I remember him, or her?

I knew that we didn't really have a dog, and that this was just a cover story Jake had provided, at *my* request, in case I had actually ended up wandering around in the wrong yard. I knew exactly why we had invented the story, but *could not access that information* in a useful way. Jake had said, "Just tell them that you are looking for *your* dog," and "Don't worry about *the* dog." Linguistically each of these implies that there *is* a dog, and having retained Jake's utterances, I could not make this "knowledge" of the mythical dog go away. In my current brittle cognitive state, because it was more current, this linguistic knowledge was interfering with my ability to access my historical knowledge that *we had no dog*.

When I found myself in novel states like this, it was important for me to figure out exactly what I did know, and exactly what I did not know. Making sense of the data from these kinds of episodes allowed me to build strategies to effectively "fake it," and thus cover up my deficits in the future. My inability to remember the dog was particularly troubling, because this was a failure I'd never encountered before, and I was now wondering whether I needed to permanently add this scenario to my stockpile of "concussion problems for which I had to be prepared." I had no strategy for working around a dog—as in, a member of my family—that was simply *gone* from my memory.

I reasoned that even if I had managed to more or less sneak into the house, surely the dog would have barked, or come to see me. I was losing coordination in my hands but I managed to press speed-dial five and call Qianwei upstairs in the house.

"Hey, Clark," she said. "When are you getting home?"

"I think maybe I already am home," I replied.

"What? What do you mean? Where are you?" she asked. I couldn't figure out how to explain.

"It's okay, sweetheart," I told her. "I'll see you soon. Say, can you tell me what our dog looks like?"

Qianwei was taken aback. "Huh?" she said. "What do you mean? We don't have a dog. Look, can I call you back? I am watching something on Chinese TV that's about to end." Then she hung up. So now, not only did *I* not remember what our dog looked like, Qianwei didn't either. This made things even harder for me to work around.

With some effort I managed to press speed-dial nine to call my daughter Nell on her cell phone. (She was downtown at a concert in Grant Park.) I reminded her that the next day was her mother's birthday, and to be sure to call. I then casually asked her what our dog looked like. Exasperated, she said, "Dad, we don't *have* a dog." So I let her get back to her concert. I found out later that her friends thought I was drunk.

This had now become a real problem. I had no clue how to work around it:

1. I did not remember the dog. And not only did I not remember the dog, but I also did not have the sense that I actually *did* remember the dog, and was just unable to make use of the information—a problem that I knew well. Instead, I had a total blank spot where the dog should have been, which was new to me.

2. I was used to relying on all sorts of cues to help me "fake" getting through difficult situations. One of my heuristics was that Jake was generally expert in all areas in which he claims knowledge. He is brilliant, extremely well informed, and precise. When I had asked Jake about the dog he had not said, "You do not have a dog," but instead had said,

"Don't worry about *the* dog." Linguistically this implies that I *had* a dog, and that I was instructed not to worry about him, or her. Jake had gotten me home. Jake was the expert.

3. Qianwei and Nell had told me we didn't have a dog, but this didn't explain away *Jake's* "dog," for which I had already formed a cognitive imprint.

4. Although completely losing all memory of *our dog* was novel, I was still used to the general problem of all kinds of strange things happening to me, wherein I had to adjust to my own deficits while at the same time mostly hiding them from others.

5. But Qianwei and Nell did not remember the dog either. How should I deal with this? I didn't know how to reconcile a world where not only did I not remember important information (or could not access it), but other people developed the same deficits as well.

It was as though I were revealing some under-the-hood construction of the universe in which other people were really me, or connected to me, in some nonphysical "we are all the same person" way—like tendons under the skin of the physical world, like Jung's collective unconscious. Examining such underpinnings of the world, and considering the structure of how it was put together, was something that I had to do all the time, just to get by. In compensating for my concussed brain, I often had to piece together reality from the kinds of detailed input that everyone else just filtered out without thought.

But this enigma was different. I just couldn't "get" it, and I couldn't let it go either. It was too important to ignore. In a downward spiral, I pressed my exhausted brain even further, forcing it to create the symbols of thought, trying to make sense of it all. In the end, out of desperation—struggling with the last of my brain power to manage the geometry of pressing speed dial six on my phone—I called Jake one last time.

"I'm sorry. I'm sorry!" I said, forming my words with difficulty. "I just can't get this dog thing, and it is so extremely unusual that I feel I have to get to the bottom of it. I fear that I am finally losing my grip on reality. Not only can't I remember anything about the dog—which would be unusual in itself—but Qianwei and Nell can't remember the dog either. Somehow I have 'infected' them with my brain damage. I don't know what to make of it."

Jake said, "Really: don't worry about it, Clark. You *don't* have a dog. We just made up the dog so that you would have a story in case it turned out to not be your house, and some old bald guy asked you what you were doing in his yard."

Jake's "You don't have a dog" contained no information that I did not already know. Nonetheless it changed my current *linguistic* knowledge of the world in a way that allowed me to access that information, and finally allowed me to sew the pieces together.

I went upstairs and fell asleep next to Erin, who was crashed out on our bed, and whom—thankfully—I *did* recognize. Qianwei came in from watching TV a few hours later, and I recognized her as well.

I was more or less normal the next morning, noticing only a distinct increase in the misuse of words when sending e-mail for my work. I was also able to reconstruct the memories of what had taken place the day before with a great deal of accuracy, and from them made these notes. Because it was such an interesting episode, I verified everything against my phone log, and by retracing my steps through the drive home.

AT LEAST WE CAN LAUGH–
PAIN AND HUMOR

There are low points with concussion, but there are amusing times as well. Here we will touch on one of the low points—concussion pain—which none of us likes to think about. But then we'll look at the other side of this life adventure too, examining one of the many bizarre episodes that ultimately were just so quirky as to be funny.

PAIN. Pain, relative to concussion, comes in three forms: the head and neck pain that comes with thinking, nausea, and the intense pain of sensory overload.

My form of head pain originated inside the top of my head and spread over the sides of my skull. Neck pain was intense, starting underneath the base of my skull and then extending down along the thick muscles that connect to my shoulders.

This neck pain was felt as an undifferentiated, throbbing ache that would not go away.

In the first months after the crash I had head pain from when I first rose in the morning until I went to bed in the evening. It often woke me up at night. Later that first year it went away—unless I had to *think*, which of course was relatively often. I went through several large bottles of ibuprofen to help with the pain, which over time led to a minor stomach ulcer.

I am lucky to be pretty good at dealing with pain. For example, I haven't bothered with dental novocaine—preferring to deal with the pain using meditative techniques—though I've had a few fillings and four dental caps over the years.

But concussion pain is significant. I learned to go to the 7-Eleven store near my house to get a large bag of ice if I was going to attempt, say, balancing my checkbook, or working out the geometry for building a dormer in my house. For certain kinds of mental challenges requiring the manipulation of symbols, such as even simple arithmetic, I would start to get nausea and head pain within about five minutes. Within ten minutes the pain was so intense that it was hard to keep going. At the twenty-minute mark, depending on the task, I would be gritting my teeth, sweating and shaking. But sometimes the work just had to get done, and I had no choice but to persist.

While I was working, I would have had the bathtub filling with cold water. When the pain got so bad that I couldn't push through it anymore, I would empty the ice into the tub, take off my clothes, and lower myself down into the ice water to freeze the muscles in my head, neck, and upper back—thus getting at least some relief. Lowering yourself into an ice bath is . . . inconvenient. And it doesn't get easier over time. But it was better than the head pain.

As discussed, the link between our bodies and the muscles that control our eyes is complex: with even a minute change in the orientation of our head we adjust our eyes to keep them stable with respect to the environment. When we think (e.g., multiply two numbers in our head, or try to recall the name of our second cousin), our eyes move in response to our thoughts. When these feedback systems, and others like them, are damaged, signals to the body may get crossed, and muscles can get knotted up.

At least some of my distress may have been caused by what later turned out to be problems with the integration of my 3D spatial hearing—which the body uses to manipulate the spine, and turn one's head toward objects that are of interest; and my 3D vision—which also places objects within the space around us and which fine-tunes movements of the spine, neck, and eye muscles to bring the object into focus. When these two systems don't agree, the signals to the muscles conflict, and, again, the muscles may get tied up in knots.

The second type of concussion pain, nausea, could be brought on by any number of things. For example, as we have seen, when I had to think about anything that required internal visualization, when I had to perform two tasks at once, or when I had to overrely on my eyes for balance, I would experience nausea. Most of the time it was my tolerance for this nausea that was the limiting factor in how long I could work.

The third kind of pain can be even more intense than the nausea, and is hard to describe to someone who has not experienced it. It comes from cognitive or sensory overload—often from unfiltered sensory input that cannot be turned off, but sometimes just from the act of thinking, which is itself, of course, a highly visual process. In my case the worst culprits were auditory input such as spoken text that demanded visualization of *meaning* as the audio stream was translated into the internal symbols of thought; complex visual patterns that had to be sorted out, such as making sense of grocery store shelves; trying to perform two or more tasks at once; and last, simply thinking about anything of even marginal complexity. In the first few months bright lights were a problem. Loud sounds—especially if they were high-pitched—were always a problem and could leave me doubled over, holding my ears. In extreme cases, overload from such relentless sensory input is torture—like having a bell lowered over your head while someone beats on it with a sledgehammer, while at the same time someone else is shining a searchlight in your eyes, and filling your nose with sulfur fumes. When this happens, the only thing you want to do is curl up and hide, or run to get away from it, in a purely primal, brain-stem way.

After recovery, and as the concussion problems went away, it became quite clear how the continual presence of pain in my life had just ground me down over time, sapping my energy and taking out some of the cheerfulness of waking up each day. I am glad to be rid of it, and my heart goes out to those with head injuries who have to deal with this in their lives.

But even if life has some challenges, it is generally better than the alternative! If we are going to consider the downsides, we should also consider, as well, the gallows *humor* that would sometimes arise from how ridiculous some of my symptoms became.

RULE FOLLOWING. Before he moved to San Diego, Jake and I would go out to eat every few weeks. In general, going out requires that many decisions be made: what time to meet, where to meet, what type of food, which restaurant, who is driving, where to park, what to order, where to sit, and so on. This is a potential nightmare for a concussive who has lost the ability to *decide*. So, knowing of my difficulties, Jake would make the decisions for both of us. I myself got in the habit of simply following rules at such times, which, to a large extent, obviated the need to make choices. For example, I might use the rule to always work from the top of the menu and order the first acceptable entree to avoid having to decide what to eat.*

One evening Jake called up. I told him I was available, so he said, "Okay, we are going to eat at *Tiffin* on Devon Avenue in Chicago. I am driving. I will pick you up at seven thirty. I will order for both of us. Be ready in an hour."

I had had a long day. My brain-batteries were drained. Consequently I intentionally placed myself in rule-following mode, to avoid getting locked up over any decisions that might arise. I would follow internal scripts, and was prepared to accept imperative commands from both Jake and myself.

Devon Avenue is the center of a large ethnic Indian neighborhood in Chicago. There are many small stores with bright displays of Indian clothes, specialty groceries, Bollywood videos, and so on. An endless slow-moving traffic jam chokes the streets, and pedestrians crowd the sidewalks. It is a visually taxing environment, and to traverse it I stuck very close to my script, which included the idea of mindlessly following all the rules of eating out.

After we had left the car and walked a block and a half

---

*Putting myself in rule-following mode worked to avoid problems with specific, highly structured scripts like going to dinner. There was, however, no algorithm that ever worked for avoiding choice in general.

toward the restaurant, I stopped in the middle of the sidewalk, frozen in place. Jake doubled back.

"Come on. What are you doing?" he asked. He was peckish, and annoyed.

"I am trying to *not* go into that store," I said, indicating one of the many stores whose windows were stacked high with cheap electronics.

"Why would you want to go in there?" he asked. Jake was understandably puzzled.

"I don't!" I said. "That's why I'm trying to not go in." I was concentrating heavily—working hard, staring intently at the store, but—except for being able to speak—still frozen in place. I nodded toward the door and said, "Look."

Jake looked up. On the door was a prominent sign that said COME IN!

"I'm trying not to go in," I said again. "I'm just able to keep from doing it, with effort, but I'm not able to make my feet go down the sidewalk."

The problem, of course, was that I was in rule-following mode, and the sign was giving me instructions: COME IN! To *not* go in, I had to violate the instructions. This was proving difficult for me to resist, and impossible for me to ignore.

"Why don't you just walk past it!" exclaimed Jake. "You're an idiot!"

"It's true," I responded. "I know exactly what is going on. I *know* that that is just a stupid sign put out to attract pedestrians into this store. I know that I don't want to go into the store. I know that all I have to do is move my feet and walk past it. I know that I am in rule-following mode so that I can get through dinner with you despite having this concussion damage. But none of that helps. I still can't move, except into the store."

As usual, I also felt guilty. But the truth of it was that, once again, there was nothing I could do. People with stage fright, or motion sickness, also understand exactly what is happening to them, but they can't stop their own symptoms from occurring either.

I started laughing at the ridiculousness of the situation, which at first annoyed the hungry Jake further—he was quite enthusiastic in his response when I suggested he give me a push. But soon he was laughing too, and I took some good-natured ribbing about it later during dinner: "What a brain-dead moron! Do you also need me to cut up your food for you?"

Once I had placed myself in rule-following mode it was difficult for me to make the transition out of it. By contrast, the healthy human brain can switch in and out of rule-following mode in the blink of an eye and with no effort whatsoever.

PROCESSING THE AUDIO SIGNAL

AUDIO SLOWNESS. One of the profound capabilities we have is turning sounds into words, words into images, and both images and words into meaning. Most of us do this effortlessly through-out the day, and at least part of the time when we are dreaming at night. If we stop to think about it, it is actually a nontrivial computation to turn, for example, the *sound* of the word "dog" (the phonemes) into the word *dog*, into an image of the written form of the word *d-o-g*, into an image of an *actual dog*, and into the conceptual *meaning* of dog-ness. Along the way we might also have picked up, from the context, that we mean *our* dog, with her attendant images, relationships, emotions, and history.

But we can perform such transformations, in all directions, without thought, seamlessly. Unless we get concussions, that is. Then the system breaks down. In the years before treatment, I became a walking laboratory for studying not only the minute details of human audio processing, but also the complex interactions between our hearing and our visual/spatial systems.

Studies in cognitive science have shown that trying to process two simultaneous aural streams at once—specifically one that is retained in memory and a live one coming in through the ears—is challenging for anyone. For concussives, who because of audio slowness may often be trying to play catch-up by buffering what was previously said and simultaneously trying to process that information along with what is currently coming in through their ears—and who are also by the way particularly stressed by doing two things at once—this is a recipe for disaster. Thus the real-time processing of speech is a serious and ubiquitous challenge for them.*

Here is how it worked:

I am listening to spoken conversation (including over a broadcast medium). I hear the first sentence, and am trying to process it in real time. But the speaker is moving too fast, and my ability to retrieve the symbolic images representing the speaker's meaning starts to lag behind. By the time the second sentence is being uttered I have not completely made sense of the first sentence. So now I have to either buffer the *sound* of the first sentence in memory briefly (a form of what is known as the *articulatory loop*) as I work through the

---

*The pathology of concussion may also contribute to this problem, especially in older concussives. Some of concussion damage is due to axonal injuries—injuries in the connections between neurons. It is believed that some axonal regeneration can take place, but that the regenerated connections may not be as efficient as before (especially in people over forty), resulting in slower processing speeds.

phonemes to figure out what they mean, or translate the sentence into an associated visual image of the words. But while I am still processing the first sentence in this way I have to simultaneously listen to the incoming sound of the second sentence being spoken.

To make matters worse, as I fall farther behind, I automatically start using *error-correction* algorithms to fill in the blanks for words that I have lost—and this is complex processing that uses up a lot of additional cognitive resources. So now we have at least *three* real-time tasks running at once: continuing to listen to the current audio stream, buffering and reviewing what was already said, and error correction on both of these interference-damaged audio streams. At this point cognitive meltdown is not far off: the size of the buffered material spirals out of control, and soon I cannot keep up.

Importantly, my ability to filter out sensory input also fails, so the incoming words can't be tuned out, and the system can't be turned off. Nor can I stop attempting to process the input, no matter how painful it becomes. Nausea sets in, and the incoming words and phrases become like little hand grenades setting off these cognitive explosions in my head. At this point social difficulties arise. The only remedies involve physical actions like hanging up the phone on someone, leaving the room, covering my ears, and begging the speaker to stop talking—social gaffes I am forced to commit many hundreds of times over the course of my injury.

I had an accurate gauge for the change in the speed of my audio processing: Prior to the crash I had no problem listening to baseball scores as reported on the radio. The announcer would read through teams and scores, usually putting the winning team first ("The Phillies, at home, beat the Reds today eleven to two"), but sometimes mixing in other reversed forms for variety ("The Giants were blanked seven to nothing by the Cards at Pac Bell Park"). Immediately images of the teams, their colors, their parks, and maybe some of their stars would come to mind. My encoding of the winning and losing teams was spatial, with the winning team higher up in my mental image than the losing team. Additionally, I placed the teams geographically, not only within a mental map of the United States, but also on the NSEW grid, relative to my own current orientation. (That is, if I happened to be facing north, I could automatically point right [east] to where the Phillies and Reds played.) Following the crash, I'd only be able to make sense of perhaps three of twelve scores, and I had no geographical grounding for any of them.

Phone conversations (which importantly take place through only one ear) were the most taxing—especially via badly digitized cell phone audio streams. Speech that additionally placed specific kinds of cognitive load on me were also difficult, such as the metaphor-filled and highly intellectual sermons given at the church I attended with my children.

SPEAKING STYLE. The speaking style of a person was also critically important in determining how hard it was for me to manage a conversation with them. My friend Mary spoke in precise, descriptive language and was easy for me to follow: "Anne, Brian, and Sarah came to my apartment at seven thirty just after I had finished dinner. We sang four madrigals by de Lassus." My friend Frank was much more of a challenge. He is smart, broadly read, and has profound reflections on many, and varied, subjects. But he tends to use imprecise language, often interspersed with ambiguous placeholders. Taken together these are a difficult combination. He might say, for example, "We were thinking about jazz groups, so I thought we should just do it. I went into the store and bought some stuff that you might like, such as Miles Davis, and I could send the thing to you." Prior to the crash, I could queue up the placeholders "do it," "stuff," and "thing," until I figured out what he was talking about. After getting the concussion, I couldn't. I would follow him up until the phrase "do it," then just lock up, waiting for a picture to emerge. In the meantime I had to queue up the ongoing audio stream of what he was saying. The multitasking required to sort it all out was often very fatiguing.

I also had two very specific difficulties in holding conversations with my mother, who lives in northern California. In the years since I left home, my mother picked up the habit of taking a bite of food, and then talking. When she talked with food in her mouth, the altered phonemes supported only approximations of the words she was speaking. Normals would have little problem apprehending her original meaning—performing natural error correction—but as a concussive I fell further and further behind in trying to parse her food-damaged speech. I was easily overwhelmed. I often had to get up from family gatherings and leave the room in a hurry, which was embarrassing for everyone.

More important, my mother has trouble retrieving nouns. She will start a sentence and then pause while she is trying to think of the label for whatever it is that she is talking about. While this problem tends to progress with age in many people, in my mother's case, somewhat ironically, this speech pattern started when she fell off a horse as a teenager, fractured her skull, and suffered a concussion. My mother might, for example, say, "I am going down this afternoon to get the . . . [long pause] . . . brakes checked on my truck."

Because of the damage to my audio processing, I was already hypervigilant about gathering in the audio stream to form it into symbols, and especially wary of symbolic "dropouts" from parts of the stream simply lost because of the slowness of my processing. During the pauses in Mom's speech—when she was searching for a label—I would work particularly hard to "fill in the blank," even though it was not intended that I do so, and even though, in most cases, there was no possible way I could.

The problem was, there were already so many things that I really *did* miss in the audio stream that I *had* to be hypervigilant: when something seemed missing, I would immediately fire off a background daemon to try to find out (a) *where* the piece of the conversation was missing, and (b) *what* it was—then have it get back to me with that information. Unfortunately, with my mother's pauses, although nothing was missing—and it would be appropriate to just wait—at an important processing level, I didn't know this; it was too similar to the ongoing instances when concussion damage did continually cause me to drop out parts of the audio stream.

The result of this cycle was fatigue. I would often reach the point of simply having to abruptly end phone conversations with her. I love my mom. She is also fascinating to talk with. (How many eighty-year-olds read a nonfiction book a day, then try to fit in their three-mile run, and a trip to the Curves gym before they go down to give a piano recital for the "old people" at the local nursing home?) It was never that I did not want to talk with her, but this was understandably not always clear to her. It is socially awkward to have to hang up the phone on your mother.

I would coach my mom to "think first, then speak" so that she would not start to talk until she had already fully retrieved everything she was going to say. This helped, and my mom was willing, but it was an ongoing problem for us—communication between one concussive and another!

JOKES. The audio stream works in both directions, of course, and in my case this highlighted an interesting phenomenon. I generally had much less difficulty *generating* speech than I did understanding it. This was most obvious when trading jokes with a group of people: I could tell jokes without much trouble, yet was often almost completely unable to understand them.

Telling jokes is a creative activity, and generative in nature. It involves memory, creativity, sensitivity to one's audience, and a sense of timing. Because concussion requires so many inventive workarounds each day, a concussive's creativity gets a lot of exercise.

Understanding jokes, on the other hand, requires deductive reasoning, and often the comparison of more than one thread of thought at the same time. It is the odd juxtaposition of these multiple threads (such as in multiple meanings in wordplay jokes), often processed within a certain time context, that make the jokes funny. In addition, a joke teller will time the delivery of the joke to match the processing speeds of her listeners.

After getting the concussion I was often not able to follow a joke, or "get" it. It turns out that the understanding of jokes is a very specific listening/brain skill.

First, as above, I would lag behind in my ability to keep up with the audio-to-symbolic translation of the input signal, and would thus lose pieces of information. But jokes typically depend on the teller giving just *exactly* the right amount of such information: give too little, and listeners do not have enough cues to work out what is odd—they miss the point; give too much and there is no suspense or moment of surprise.

Second, I was not able to process more than one piece of information at a time, and even if I did catch up, it was not with the natural timing that a normal would use. When the timing is thrown off in this way, and the abstract double-meaning information that has to be just hinted at in the right way is missed, the joke is difficult to understand. If the revealing of a double meaning is made at the wrong time, a joke is not funny.

So when friends and family would gather around after a meal and tell jokes, I might tell a good joke of my own, then spend the rest of the time tuning out, smiling when others smiled, and laughing when others laughed—but I mostly didn't have a clue what they were talking about. The following table illustrates how a damaged audio stream can particularly affect the understanding of jokes:

WHAT I HEARD	WHAT THE KID SAID
What do you eat . . . watching movies?	What do you eat when you are watching horror movies?
. . . *Dessert!*	. . . *I scream!*
What do you eat . . . horror movies . . . computers?	What do you eat when you are watching horror movies about computers?
. . . *Potato chips!*	. . . *Chips!*

SOCIAL CHALLENGES

A concussive's life is socially complex. In general, people won't understand what a concussive's limitations are. There are a number of reasons for this: Many concussives will not, themselves, fully understand what has happened to them. Those who do may very well be attempting to hide their symptoms from others anyway—trying to restore as much normalcy to their lives as they can. Then there is the strange feature—disconcerting to others—of the concussive being almost completely normal one moment, and then quite incapacitated a few minutes later.

It was my common experience that people—including both those who knew me well and strangers—saw my concussion symptoms as just *weird*, and also, in some global way, *annoying*. To be honest, their reactions were probably quite reasonable: my symptoms *were* weird, and often caused me to act in ways that under normal circumstances would be inexplicable. It was often difficult, if not impossible, to explain to others what was happening to me. People were naturally likely to account for my behavior in the way that made the most sense to them—that I was drunk, that I was difficult, that I was rude. Of course, that's what we all do—we try to explain the world by using what we know of it. Unfortunately this led to repercussions in my life—some of them bizarre.

RAMON'S BRAKES. One day, I was playing baseball with my son in the front yard. Predicting the visual path of the white baseball—against a backdrop of bright green leaves shimmering in the sunlight—was fatiguing. My cognitive and sensory filters were breaking down. But my son had just started playing in Little League, and I knew it was very important to him to practice, so I forced myself to push through my discomfort.

As we were playing, Ramon, an older man from the neighborhood—a casual friend of mine who would sometimes come by to talk about politics and neighborhood concerns— pulled his car up next to me to tell me that he wanted me to trim my bushes at the corner of the alley. His eyesight was starting to decline, and my bushes further impaired his view when he made the turn into the street. Unfortunately, his old car had terribly squeaky disc brakes. Because of my phonosensitivity I keeled over onto the street in fetal position, covering my ears to shield them from the painful screeching sound, before I could hear what he had to say. He got mad and drove off. Variations of this same difficult episode happened twice more that same week, and the last two times Ramon was yelling at me as he drove off. I made a mental note to go over to his house on the weekend and ask him what had been on his mind.

But I was too late. Ramon got up early on Saturday morning and cut down all of the young trees I had been cultivating for five years along the side of my yard, which had nothing to do with the bushes at the end of the alley. When I noticed what he was doing, and leaned out the window to ask him to stop, he shouted insults at me at the top of his lungs for my children and neighbors to hear.

I later went to his house to talk to him. After getting him to calm down, and apologizing about the bushes, I asked him why he was so angry—surely those bushes, which we both agreed hadn't reached a sight-impairing point yet, couldn't have been enough to make him cut down my trees and scream obscenities at me!

His face got red. You could see he was getting mad all over again, though he kept it in check because his wife was there.

"You started it!" he accused. "Why did you have to be so rude? I kept my cool that first time you made such a big deal of not listening to me, covering your ears, and lying in the street like a big baby, in front of your boy. I never saw such a thing! The second time you did it I couldn't believe it. Who the hell acts like that, like a spoiled little kid, closing your eyes, covering your ears? What did I ever do to *you* that it is so important you can't take three minutes to listen to what I have to say? The third time on Friday was too much. I decided to teach you a lesson. You're an asshole, is the thing. I guess, what did you expect?"

Even though he listened—suspiciously—as I tried to explain about the brain damage and the squealing brakes, he didn't really get it. He pointed out that I seemed fine when I was tossing the baseball to my son, and although in the end he apologized about the trees, it was obvious he didn't quite believe me. By now I could easily recognize the half-glazed, half-skeptical look that meant I was being given a little leeway, but no real understanding. Despite the mutual apologies, after that he was no longer friendly toward me when we'd see each other around the neighborhood.

Ramon was a grumpy old guy, sure. But in many ways he was a good man, and someone that I respected for his life of both conviction and action, which I knew about from the chats we used to have. It was not pleasant for either of us to have this friendship end so badly—another casualty of the concussion.

SCANNER BEEP. At Food 4 Less, a local grocery store, I often had trouble with the loud *beep* from the checkout scanners after the difficult visual pattern matching required when shopping for food. When I asked clerks to turn down the volume, they would generally look at me like I was nuts, and refuse. The problem was that I could not load my groceries on the belt when the clerk was scanning other items, because I had to use my hands to cover my ears. I also could not bag my groceries if the clerk started scanning the groceries of the person after me in line, using the alternate bagging area.*

One evening—after I'd gone without food for several days because I'd had to abort two previous shopping trips due to debilitating concussion problems—I was in the checkout line

---

*I tried wearing earplugs when shopping but the change in the aural environment was usually too disconcerting. It also further overloaded my visual system, which had to make up for the loss of environmental *spatial context* information I ordinarily got from my ears.

at Food 4 Less and again having trouble with the scanner beep. I was getting desperate, and because I just couldn't make the clerk understand my situation, I finally refused to swipe my credit card until I had my groceries bagged: if the clerk started scanning the groceries of the next customer I would not be able to finish bagging my own. Each *beep!* caused me to double over with pain. My motor coordination had deteriorated, and I was on edge because I knew everyone was waiting as I labored in slow motion with my groceries.

When I finally got outside—it was hard to move my feet—I could make no sense of the parking lot. While I was standing there wondering where my car might be, and how I could find it, *Bang!* My shoulder exploded in pain. I spun around to see the very angry face of the man who had waited behind me in line—he had punched me in the shoulder. His fist was cocked again, and it looked as though he was now going to hit me in the head. Instead he yelled something in Spanish, then walked away.

One afternoon the following August, I was again debilitated from food shopping, and had given up after buying just a few essential items that I was now carrying with me. I was walking in slow motion back to my car in the parking lot: left foot, right foot, trying to make sense of the visual scene around me. A young professional woman walked briskly past me and got in her big SUV, parked a short way down the parking aisle. She jerked back two feet, the way people do when they are in a hurry, moving her SUV out to get a better view and to alert others that she was backing up, before finishing the arc of her backward turn into the aisle. But I was now directly opposite her car. She looked me in the eye in her large side-view mirror. When she saw that I was walking slowly she glared at me, then started mouthing angry words—I guess thinking I was "slow-walking" on purpose, just to be annoying. She jammed on the accelerator pedal and as the car shot toward me, I just managed to jump out of the way, sprawling on the hot pavement, with my groceries flying in all directions. She then sped away, tires screeching. This was yet another case of "brain tax," the social penalty of concussion: A woman got mad because I was not acting normal. She assumed I was being aggressive and adversarial, and responded in kind.*

LECTURES. There were social aspects of my job that were troublesome as well. For example, attending academic lectures was a necessary part of my work as a professor but quite treacherous for me.

In a typical scene, several years after the crash, I attended a job talk for a vacant faculty position. I was following Power-Point slides along with twenty-five of my colleagues. Ten minutes into the talk, *audio slowness* set in, and I began to lose my ability to filter out unwanted sensory information. In addition to forming the complex mental images representing the new research being presented, I was also constructing the judgment that for technical reasons this lecture was not very well formed—and this was important because it was a job talk, and I'd later be called on to decide whether this candidate would be a good teacher.

---

*This was an instance of "emergency adrenal mode" where I called on extreme resources to respond to special circumstances. But it took its toll: Several people helped me to my car, with my groceries. I waited for a long time before I could drive. I had to leave the groceries in the car when I got home—where they spoiled several days later. I went without food the rest of the week.

Taken all together, my limited cognitive resources were rapidly draining away. I had to time this just right. I needed to stay as long as I could manage, because assessing these candidates was part of my job. But if I stayed too long, I'd be unable to get out of the room without causing a disturbance—an uncomfortable faux pas given how important this talk would be for the candidate. It would be bad if I had to stop the lecture and ask someone to help me from the room. It would be almost as bad if I had to cover my ears and stagger out on my own.

The problem was the cognitive overload from my having to manage so many independent symbolic streams of thought, and my inability to filter out the unwanted sensory input. I'd hear words from the speaker; I'd hear words the speaker had already said but which were still queued up for processing; I'd hear the squeak of a chair next to me; I'd see candidate words for audio error correction in front of my eyes; I'd hear myself judging the candidate's teaching abilities; I'd be rewriting the slides the way *I* would have done it for clarity; I'd see shadows on the floor; I'd see color patches of clothes; I'd hear the tick of the wall clock, and so on. I'd soon be managing head pain, and nausea, and trying to keep my balance in my chair. But I couldn't stop any of the processing, or shut out any of the raw input.

Over time I grew crafty at managing such lectures. I'd sit in the back where I could surreptitiously put in industrial earplugs, and close my eyes, to get a break from the sensory input. I'd make sure to be near a wall so that I could hold on to it for balance as I snuck out. If a video was available I could watch it later. I'd try to let the speaker know ahead of time that I would not be able to stay for the whole lecture.

In general, if I was rested I could manage about twenty-five minutes of a lecture before reaching the danger zone when I could no longer walk.

ODD JUXTAPOSITIONS. Besides the constant worry that I'd have to explain myself to others or risk seriously offending them, there was the added concern that some malicious person would use this information to take advantage of my defenselessness. And I did encounter such people in my life. I had to be always alert, though I often could not understand exactly how I was being exploited, and could not form any real plan to protect myself. At the same time, the only way for me to survive *in general* was to give in, and, at those times of almost childlike helplessness, blindly trust others to help me get by. This juxtaposition was complex for me emotionally as well as cerebrally: a mixture of trusting, acceptance, and a hoped-for recovery on the one hand; and of watchfulness, unrelenting vigilance, and helplessness on the other.

Additionally, everyone, including me, had trouble figuring out my place when I was to cooperate with others: could I be trusted to get the job done? As a high-functioning concussive I had this strange aspect to my life: On the one hand I was helpless and rather stupid—unable, for example, to manage even the simplest kind of planning. On the other hand, I was performing brilliantly, and with stunning creativity, from the moment I woke up until the moment I fell asleep—just to find a way to get through a normal day. In the end I became reluctant to make commitments, something that may be common among concussives.

STUCK IN THE MOMENT OF IMPACT. When visiting Jake in San Diego, I happened to read a book by John Conroy that he had on his shelf, about victims of torture in the seventies and eighties. Among other topics, the book raises the issue of the long-term effects of torture, based on interviews with victims. Our cultures and our lives were very different, yet I felt a strong, elemental kinship with those victims on a human level that led to an arresting epiphany.

Although my experience was certainly nothing like what these survivors had had to endure, it struck me how much we nonetheless shared in one very particular aspect of our lives: in one important way, the voices in this book spoke for me as well. In the cases covered in the book, the torture had been exposed, and those responsible had been found accountable, at least by the public. The story had come out.

This was, of course, important and cathartic for the survivors, after all the years of living with public denials of their horrific experience. But then a strange thing happened. The hubbub died down. Everyone seemed to agree that the problem had at last been handled. Everyone else moved on, including the torturers themselves.

But the survivors did not.

Despite the social acknowledgment of their suffering, and a resultant lessening of their outrage, the *neurological trauma* was still with them just as strongly as before, and something they had to deal with every hour, and every minute, of both their waking and sleeping lives.

I often felt that way too: the rest of the world had wrapped my brain damage up in a neat little explainable package and moved on . . . but very deep down, in the lowest level of my neural programming, *I hadn't*. Neurologically, traumatically, I was still stuck back in that moment of impact in September 1999.

The fact of my much later stunning recovery, which included being freed from the imprint of the original trauma, suggests to me that such dual treatments as I underwent—each of which, as we'll soon see, addresses deeply elemental features of *cognition*—might similarly help victims of deep *emotional* trauma, which can itself cause physical and neurological traumatic injury to the brain. Perhaps they could then move on too.

PHYSICAL CHANGES

SENSORY FILTERS. All input and output from our brains takes place through the medium of our bodies, and thus the two are highly integrated. In some views they are inseparable. But with concussion the relationship between the brain and the body can change, and for the concussive there may be many unusual and disconcerting experiences as a result.

One common experience I had was that under cognitive stress my *sensory filters* would change. These filters have two main jobs. First, they operate to exclude most of the potential input because it is not of interest to us. Second, they chunk together pieces of the remaining input into *meaning*. Additionally, these two processes work together: In a greatly simplified version we might imagine there are twenty layers of such filters. At each level the filtered and concentrated input signal is passed upward toward the rest of the brain—gathering meaning along the way. But at the same time signals are also sent back downward (toward the original body sensors) to further bias the way the previous layer applies its filtering. In this way we get raw input from the bottom up, but also, at the same time, a continuous stream of biasing information helping us to "know what to look for or listen to" that is passed back from the top down. In this way we eliminate increasing portions of the incoming signal as irrelevant to the context and meaning we have now partially determined.*

The brain also works with the extended body to control the process of gathering input information by changing our posture orientation, by changing the properties of our eyes (including, e.g., the balance between the different retinal systems), by affecting the level of our physical arousal, of our hormone balance, and so on, each of which affects how we appraise the world.

Consider, for example, the following "London in the rain" exercise. I wrote it on the whiteboard in one of my undergraduate AI classrooms before the students arrived, then asked them during the lecture what it said:

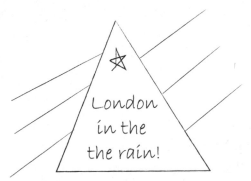

Figure 1: London in the rain!

---

*Surprisingly, modern research has shown that there are significantly more neural pathways dedicated to top-down feedback control than there are for the actual bottom-up feed-forward input signal that they are filtering.

Naturally they told me that it said "London in the rain." When I asked them again to tell me what it *really* said, they replied, "London in the rain." At the end of fifteen minutes of this, my forty students were ready to lynch me, and to avoid a mutiny I had to manually explain their mistake. (Carefully count the words in the illustration, pointing to them with your finger.) They literally *couldn't see* the words in front of them.

In this case, subliminal error correction in the students' brains altered their perception, and probably yours as well—a sensory filter. This is an example of our brains chunking together small bits of information to form *meaning* under control of what our brains are expecting to see.

After suffering the concussion, at times of brain fatigue, I often lost efficacy in my sensory filters. As we have seen, I would, instead, get a flood of sensory information—bits and pieces of the world—with no gestalt meaning attached. I had to construct meaning manually, putting together raw pieces of information, such as shapes and colors and the sounds that came with them, to make sense of the world around me.

BODY-SENSE COGNITION AND BRAIN FLU. At other times, because of impoverished visual and balance systems, I would need to rely on my *body feelings* partly as a way of constructing the internal symbols of thought. When I couldn't *see* meaning in the input, I would *feel* it instead. This is difficult to describe, because it is not normally something we think about, and understanding it is also not intuitive. Yet it was an important mechanism that helped me reason about the world, and a capability that we all probably use to a lesser degree without realizing it.

Let's imagine that I ordinarily have a visual/geometric representation of the concept *conflict:* say (for simplicity's sake) *The*

Blue Team on the left, pushing and tugging against *The Red Team* on the right, one side against the other. But on this day, because of visual system fatigue I've lost the ability to *see* this concept. But my body and emotion system are functioning as normal. Now, to make up for my internal visual deficits I substitute the much more abstract emotion concepts of *pathos, desire, feeling of accomplishment*, and so on, which I can still clearly experience as felt emotions in my body. These can be combined in various ways to represent conflict: if *Blue* and *Red* both *desire* the goal *G*, and Blue *feels pathos* when Red *gets (accomplishes) the goal* *G* . . . then they are in *conflict*. In this way I could use body representations to manipulate the logic relative to *conflict* in place of the internal visual symbols that had deserted me. In the general case, *I could use body information to reason about the world.*

As a concussive, I used this sense of my body all day long— to check my surroundings, to arrange for remedial help with balance, to substitute for other kinds of symbolic representations that I could no longer map to problems in the real world, and so on. But when I got a cold, or was fatigued and sore from a hard run, my body sense changed, and this presented cognitive difficulties.

To illustrate, let's further imagine that I am grading papers for class, but on this day I have a cold. After finishing a few papers, I am losing the ability to visualize internal concepts, including *conflict*. But now, because of the cold, my body already feels feverish, which is similar to the feeling for *pathos*, and I am no longer able to feel the emotion in the usual way. But having lost pathos, I have also lost *conflict*, and without conflict I can't understand the phrase ". . . the conflict between using the most efficient algorithm, and the one that is least suscepti-ble to failure" in some graduate student's homework.

Getting a cold or the flu thus not only was a physical prob-lem, as it would be for normals, but also was attendant with the much more taxing cognitive difficulties engendered by losing many backup mechanisms for forming the symbols of thought that would get me through the day.

Perhaps it helps to think of it this way: my cognitive/sensory landscape was often a changing and unfamiliar environment, without inherent symbolic *meaning*, and requiring much thought to figure out. By contrast, my body state was relatively constant, and I was thus generally able to use this grounded propriocep-tive sense, and other body feelings, to form nonvisual symbols that still allowed reasoning and problem solving to take place. But when I lost the grounding of my body sense because of ill-ness or physical fatigue, I could no longer form these nonvisual symbols in the usual way. My internal landscape became just as unfamiliar as the unfiltered external sensory stream was.

This can be a perplexing weakness. It often left me asking myself, "What is *wrong* with me? Why am I so incapacitated by a simple cold?"

SEIZURES AND OTHER STRANGE PHENOMENA. When some-one gets a concussion there may be odd physical failures that can occur in addition to the cognitive changes, and I experi-enced a few of them myself.

Under certain kinds of cognitive loads that involved my making sense of *lines*—especially parallel or concentric lines, and also in some cases geometric rotations of shapes that had well-defined edges that could be perceived as lines—I would start having mild brain seizures that caused my whole body to shake from side to side. Here is an episode from my notes that illustrates how this would happen:

> *September 2004:* Several days ago I had a large photocopying job that I had to complete before the day was out. I was at the UPS store doing my best to keep the various piles of originals from getting mixed up. It was a complex job, entailing sorting and copying collections of documents, translating two-sided originals into one-sided copies, and so on. The intense visual appraisals required for the mental rotations—top-to-bottom, front-to-back—soon left me disoriented. Because I had a hard deadline, I had to draw extensively on my deep cognitive batteries and keep going—no matter how I felt. There were other customers waiting behind me, adding social pressure.
>
> Because of the *geometric* visual demands, I started to experience tremors that caused my whole upper body to shake back and forth. It was embarrassing to hear the "flap! flap! flap!" of the papers waving around as I worked. I kept going, and finished the job because I had to, but it was startling for others in the copy shop to watch—the shop owner offered to call an ambulance for me—and it was a real struggle for me to get home afterward. The seizure movements tapered off and finally stopped after three days.

I experienced these seizures to one degree or another about thirty times, and always with visual triggers—although it was some time before I made this connection. They lasted from a few hours to a few days. I was often afraid that these were precursors of an impending neurological collapse, but in the end, with rest, they always went away. I didn't want to take any chances with them, and when I began experiencing seizures I took this as a sign that I had to let virtually everything else go.

In March 2008, at which point I was well into my recovery, I was more confident, and my scientific curiosity took over. I found that if I tried to mimic the seizure movement manually, I could only approximate it, and I would get tired in only a minute or two. By contrast when the seizures came over me from geometric triggers, they might last for days and I wouldn't feel any muscle fatigue at all. With experimentation—at times of relatively low stress—I found that just by drawing concentric circles on a sheet of paper I could trigger an episode in as little as four minutes. I would draw a small circle, then another around it, and another around that one, up to five or six concentric circles. Then I'd start another design next to it. For variation I might mix in concentric squares.

After two horizontal rows of designs (ninety seconds) I started to feel the effects, and also as though I were "falling into" the shapes when I looked at them. After half a page of designs, if I stood up, and relaxed, I would have the seizures, and they would last for about twenty minutes.

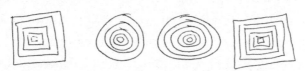

Figure 2: Hand-Drawn Concentric Circles and Squares

I was able to function well—talk, grasp things, etc.—but I had to be careful not to drop items or knock them off counters or a table top when I was picking them up. My walk was affected: I sort of stumped along, straightening my knees more than usual at the extension point, flinging my feet forward, instead of stepping.

My intuition is that if I pushed myself, say by drawing five or six pages of concentric designs, the tremors would last for several days.

Another brain-wiring problem—and the scariest one—came from a surprising source: itching.

Sometime after the car crash I realized that I could no longer effectively locate where certain kinds of back itches were, and without my being able to scratch them, they would not go away. I could feel where the itch was *supposed* to be on my back, but scratching there didn't relieve the itch. Instead I had to generally scratch all over my back, my shoulders, and my upper arms, and sooner or later the itch would gradually recede. But for this kind of itch there was never a sense of finding "the" spot. I never actually relieved the itch directly, by scratching, which is, in itself, unpleasant. (Think of a sneeze that just fades away.)

This may seem like a small problem, but I have many times thanked my lucky stars that I have at least been able to get the itch to slowly go away by scratching everywhere. What a maddening—and even potentially catastrophic—thing it would be if my random scratching were not able to get this phantom back itch to stop! To give some context about how serious this can be, consider the case in which another sufferer of a phantom itch went almost mad, and indeed ultimately scratched through not only her scalp but also her skull bone and into her brain trying to get relief from an incessant itch that she could not control.*

On one occasion, in August 2001, I temporarily lost part of my vision. I had gone to a carnival with my sister's family and my kids. I was reluctant to go on any rides where there were g-forces other than normal because of my balance problems, but on this occasion there was social pressure to go on a roller coaster so that one of the kids—who needed an accompanying adult—could go. Against my better judgment I went on the ride with him.

Afterward I lost the vision in my right eye. It was not that my eye went black, but rather that I simply could not process any information from it. I couldn't see at all, and my head hurt in a way that I'd not experienced before. This was scary. My vision was gone long enough that I feared it was going to be permanent. Fortunately, about an hour later it came back and the headache gradually receded.

RUNNING: HOW THE BODY FOLLOWS THE BRAIN. The notes on my marathon running during this period yield some unique supporting data for the power of *visualization* in controlling our lives and our bodies. I believe this has far-reaching implications.

To set the context for understanding why my own experience was important we can consider the thesis of Timothy Gallwey's book *The Inner Game of Tennis*.† In it, he talks about

---

*Atul Gawande, "The Itch," *New Yorker*, June 30, 2008 (http://www.newyorker.com/reporting/2008/06/30/080630fa_fact_gawande).
†W. Timothy Gallwey, *The Inner Game of Tennis: The Classic Guide to the Mental Side of Peak Performance* (Random House, 1974).

the idea of *seeing* oneself succeed as being the most important component of improving one's game. Similarly, in numerous interviews with sports stars like Michael Jordan and Jack Nicklaus, we find the ubiquitous idea of forming a strong mental picture of one's goals, and then *mentally rehearsing* the goals to supplement the actual physical training that takes place.

I began running in 2001, two years after the crash. I thought that perhaps if I could keep in good physical condition I would improve the blood flow to my brain, and give myself the best chance at recovery. By this time I had for two years already had little choice but to force myself to walk daily. But the forcing was highly symbolic in nature: there was nothing wrong with my legs. Rather it was the low-level "seeing" of my progress toward a destination that was diminished, and it was this visualization—the driving engine of motion—that got such a vigorous daily workout.*

But this discipline of forcing my legs to go, ignoring fatigue, strongly visualizing my goal, and persisting toward it no matter what, were activities shared with long-distance runners. They were training hard, and daily, to run marathons; I was training hard, and daily, just to get across the room, down the hall, across the parking lot.

Once I started to run, it turned out that with only minimal physical training I could run long distances. I am absolutely certain that the daily grind I went through, sometimes even

---

*You can see the strong link between the brain's visual/spatial processing and locomotion in the following way: Next time you are able to go running (or some equivalent), push yourself to where you can just keep up the pace—you are working hard. Now, try solving simple arithmetic or logic problems in your head. You'll find it is *really* hard to do both at the same time. You'll want to stop running, or drop into a more automatic pace, so that you can work out the problem in your head, because each of these tasks is competing for the same visual/spatial resources.

working against extreme debilitation to do so, year after year, prepared my brain-body system to run what ultimately became marathons.

The effect of such mental training is strong. Because of my child-care responsibilities, and my work, I had very little time to myself. I ran only when I could, and only casually—never more than twice a week, and usually far less. Yet there are many examples of the results of my ubiquitous daily *mental* exercise. For instance, in the fall of 2003 I found myself with an unheard-of Saturday morning when I didn't have any children with me, so I just ran until I felt like stopping—eight hours and *forty-one miles* later. In another example, in 2007, in the seven-month period from January through July, I was able to run only four times, for three miles or less, adding a single longer run in each of August and September. Then I completed the twenty-six-mile Chicago Marathon a few weeks later.* In all I completed marathon distances or greater twelve times during my eight years in the concussion soup. My "training" was exceedingly casual, yet my experience when running was just like my normal day: *left foot, right foot, keep going!*

---

*The race was aborted because of the extreme heat, and my path thus cut short, but I ran for an hour in Grant Park afterward and completed thirty miles.

SPIRALING DOWNWARD

MEDICAL DEAD END. My difficult experiences in the hospital notwithstanding, I made determined efforts to get the best help possible. But over the years I lost hope that the medical community had anything to offer.

By my third year after the crash, I had had appointments with two of the leading neurologists in the Chicago area. One was the consulting neurologist on a huge contract for an internationally famous sports star, which had recently been finalized only after he gave his okay regarding lingering concussion symptoms. Among his other clients were national household names in the sports world. He was compassionate about my condition. At least he understood my symptoms! The other leading neurologist diagnosed, and explained, some of my vestibular difficulties, though he asked no questions, and in the end had little else to say. Their assessment: Concussives never really get better. The brain is permanently damaged. There is often terraced improvement after three weeks, after six months, after a year, and sometimes at two years. Beyond that, no one improves. I should develop strategies for living with my permanently diminished abilities.

I went through an expensive set of tests at a highly ranked rehabilitation center. But once again, in my strongest opinion, the tests were inappropriate for concussion. In a repeat of my visit to the first neurologist (a few weeks after the crash), I managed to score in the highest percentiles on several cognition tests, but afterward I had trouble talking, and could not walk. My hands didn't work. I was in pain from the simple mental exercises. My sensory filters were failing. When I mentioned my symptoms, I was told brusquely, "That's not part of the data."

None of what I felt were the interesting components of cognitive breakdown were assessed. And, if the tests were to have been repeated, I would have scored near the bottom. When I mentioned this, I was again told that that, too, was irrelevant. There was zero accounting for changes in cognition under brain stress, which of course is one of the hallmarks of concussion.

Furthermore, there was no accounting whatsoever for differing *baseline levels* of cognitive performance from patient to patient; though I still scored very high on the mental manipulation exams relative to the average, I struggled with the exams, and they were much harder for me than they would have been prior to getting the concussion. None of this was taken into account.*

---

*Another difficulty that concussives may encounter is that there is no accounting for the interaction between independent tests: For example, a concussive is given a pattern

Despite the high cost of the tests, the institution's computers were old and the software for testing even older, running on long-outdated operating systems. I once again had the distinct impression that because there was no treatment for concussion, it was not of interest to the medical community, and concussion research did not attract much funding.

The result: I was suffering from post-concussion syndrome, legally classified as an *impairment*, not a *disability*. There wasn't much to be done. Sometimes taking a selective serotonin reuptake inhibitor (SSRI) like Prozac could help to jump-start the brain. (It didn't—no effect.)

STRESS. At the time of the crash I had worked ahead in my professional life—preparing my courses well in advance—to clear the year for research. I was also feeling good about my personal life, my first wife and I having finally ended a long-troubled marriage four months earlier. Nonetheless, even with such a clear schedule, I was now almost completely unable to keep up with my commitments. I had always been the guy who did whatever it took to get the job done—*always*—and for the longest time I still expected to wake up the next morning and be myself. I couldn't conceive of what was wrong with me, and I held myself to the same standards as always. I had no interest in considering my injury—I just wanted to get back to the work of my life. It was stressful, and frustrating for me to watch, as I had to let one thing after another go.

---

matching test on which she scores almost perfectly, but which leaves her incapacitated after only a few minutes. Following this she is given an independent test of memory on which she scores poorly because she is worn out from the first test, but which would ordinarily be no problem at all. In the classic case she'll try to explain this to the neurologist administering the tests and be dismissed because it "is not part of the tests."

After six weeks I finally realized that maybe I needed "a little more rest for a while" until I could figure out what was going on. I still had no clue what having a concussion meant, but I did intentionally adopt some different patterns in my life, and was willing to temporarily give up on many of my goals. I started to think, from time to time, "Well, I just can't get that done, so I might as well not worry about it." I stopped returning *all* my e-mail messages, I accepted losing money from incorrect charges on my phone bill, and I gave up trying to remember everyone's birthday.

Then, one day, sitting in my living room two years after the crash, once again unable to get up from my chair, I realized that I was *never going to get any better.* I recall thinking explicitly that my life had been pretty good; if I was able to get anything more from the shell that was left I would consider it serendipity. I thought about how gracefully my own father had faced his death, and had a small "ah-ha!" moment realizing that I too was now able to manage my own "partial death" in the same way.

"This is it," I reflected. "I am never going to have another normal day, or hour, or ten-minute period again. I am never going to be a real human being again. I am never going to be close to God again. I won't be publishing my research, and at some point I am going to lose my job. I'll never be able to study music again, or even organize my records so that I can listen to them."

In that moment, I just let go. I accepted that life as I had known it was over. But this explicitly did not mean that I was giving up. In fact, in a baroque way it was the opposite of giving up. Rather it was a *giving in*—a complete reorganization of how I felt about my time on earth.

So I stopped beating my head against the wall. I openly

told people that I could not handle many of their requests, and was not going to try. I set limits on what people could ask of me, and I learned to say "no" to myself for anything frivolous that would take more than a few minutes. I focused entirely on the needs of my children and on my work.

This had consequences. For example, I couldn't manage the one-eared, digitized sequence-processing component of voicemail. So I turned it off. Many people considered this a rude outrage: they wanted to be able to leave me messages, and accused me of being purposely difficult. But I knew there was nothing I could do about any of it. The *letting go* afforded me a great lessening of stress, and a relief from responsibilities that I could no longer meet.

By continuing to be deliberate about limiting my responsibilities, in the years following I gained back just enough functionality to maintain the status quo. And then in 2004, another baby (Erin) came into our lives. The obligation of being a parent to this young child—which ultimately fell almost entirely on my shoulders—required that I push myself to the absolute limit.

THE TALKING GIRL. By 2006 I was a de facto full-time single parent of my three daughters, including, most notably, two-year-old Erin, and in addition shared the custody of my son Paul, who was then eleven. It was during this period, starting seven years after the crash, that caring for Erin, and in particular attending to her developing *verbal* needs, brought me to the brink of a complete breakdown.

As any parent knows, raising children can be fatiguing. In addition, one parent alone, taking care of several children, especially while working full-time, has an increased burden. As a single parent, I was busy, and tired in the normal way, as would be expected from responding to the continual demands. But kids are dynamic too, and being genetically and culturally programmed to respond to the needs of families, mine were also able to adapt to my infirmities. So in general, we got by. If, for example, Nell needed help with her homework assignment, I would stay up late at night working on it, possibly over the course of a few days, and leave explanatory notes for her to read in the morning. But I had constraints too: I could not be counted on to drop whatever I was doing to work on a math problem for ten minutes, because the symbolic processing needed for that ten minutes might mean that I would then not be able to cook dinner.

But two-year-olds are different. Yes, they can also adapt, but the scope of their adaptations is limited. They tend to need what they need *right now*, and are not good at longer-term planning, or at waiting.

Yet even the constant demands of a two-year-old were something that, except for one issue, I could deal with. I had, after all, done it three times before. Healthy two-year-olds, while not being able to plan well for themselves, are also generally predictable, and thus random entities around which a crafty adult can himself plan: if a two-year-old is coming home from the babysitter's house where they have had several hours of play, then, no matter what their apparent mood is, the rule is they need food, and hugs, immediately—otherwise, watch out. If you want them to learn to clean up after themselves, then you have to do it with them often, and they will copy you, as play. And so on.

Basic two-year-old behavior was not the problem.

The one area, however, that was beyond Erin's control, and mine, was her essential biological and cognitive need to *talk all the time*—which in her case was also idiosyncratically emphasized. Erin was, and is, a bright, inquisitive, *engaged* girl. She is highly social, and thinking all the time, and it was also her natural toddler disposition that if a thought came into her head it was also coming out of her mouth.

The verbal style of very young children requires us to use a unique set of resources to process what they are saying. They ask questions and make pronouncements in the middle of other conversations. Their speech is often broken, and slowly formed, with many garden-path sentences that are later back-tracked and started again—especially when they are working out complex structures, as bright children are wont to do. It is as though they are thinking out loud, and the sound of their words helps them to form their ideas. For me, following this kind of communication structure was particularly taxing—as we've already seen, people's speaking styles made a big difference in how rapidly I grew fatigued.

When Erin was talking, I fell into the familiar trap of being unable to filter out the verbal/audio stream coming in through my ears: the sensory input was going to be presented to my brain whether I wanted it to be or not, and I would automatically attempt to turn her words into symbolic meaning. *Always*. It was a process beyond my control. I would then fall prey to another familiar problem: having to perform two tasks at once—in this case, making sense of what Erin was saying, and trying to do virtually anything else. In a disastrous spiral I would fall farther and farther behind as I tried to turn her constant stream of words into meaning, and also go about the rest of my life.

Here is a diary entry giving an example of Erin's speech that I was parsing throughout the day:

> "Dad . . . why do spiders like to bite people? *Do* spiders like to bite people? We have spiders in the house. I saw one. Does *that* spider *there* like to bite people? One time . . . Daddy, one time there was a spider on Mommy's sweater. *Was* that spider going to bite her? It was black. Not the sweater. The sweater was her red sweater . . . Looks nice! Was it going to bite her? Do we taste good? Like chocolate? Hey Dad. Daddy! Daddy! Can we have some strawberries? Can you get me some strawberries? Hey Dad, did you get Paul a towel with different colors too? Is that Paul's new towel? Is that like a rainbow? . . . or is it just striped different colors?"*

It was this simple combination—my inability to filter out or process spoken dialogue in real time, and Erin's continual need to talk—that almost led to a final, catastrophic meltdown. The daily processing demands of this problem just led me, over the months, to deep, deep brain fatigue.†

---

*This passage was actually recorded when Erin was slightly older, but it is representative of the earlier time.

†A scheme we worked out together was the only thing that allowed me to keep going during this period: Each morning, for more than two years, we would put on music—symphonies, string quartets, piano concertos, jazz, operas—and dance for forty minutes. Then we'd listen for another two hours during which time I would work on my computer and Erin would either continue to dance or sit quietly at her own desk and paint.

After a year and a half of this verbal explosion, I had reached the end of the line. This was a tricky place. It was not an option to *not* be taking care of Erin. She needed me as the reliable caretaking parent that she had had all her life. Her mother was, by this time, seldom at home, and additionally spending a good part of the year on business trips in China. There was not enough money for me to hire a regular babysitter—my salary already went to support two households. Yet I could no longer manage working and caring for Erin on my own. I was still, albeit in a much-reduced capacity, trying to be the guy who could be a professor, take care of everyone, raise a young child on my own, build a house on the side—the guy that always came through. *But that guy was gone.*

I had to face reality. I couldn't keep up anymore. Unless something changed, I was going to have to resign from my job, which in turn would mean losing my house, losing my ability to support my family, losing everyone's medical insurance, and likely losing contact with my older children. After so many efforts that had done nothing but further drain my resources, I had little hope of finding any help. Nonetheless, because I was now on the precipice, I was prompted to make one last-ditch effort.

It was at this point, in January 2008, that I pulled out my last remaining emergency savings and hired my second professional organizer, Heather. Heather's first task was to help me to write up a detailed letter and send it to twenty selected researchers and centers that focused on traumatic brain injury, and that might either help me themselves, or know of someone who could. We especially focused on those whose work embraced the modern idea of *brain plasticity*. But we had no luck.

In fact, over the months following, we got back only a single short response that said in effect, "I'm sorry! I can't help you at the moment, but I'll think about it." Outside of that, the silence, as always, was deafening.*

So now what?

It turned out that Heather was (and still is!) a most completely excellent devout Buddhist person, around whom good things always seem to happen to others. A while after our sending the letters Heather ran into a woman at a party who had been to see a local cognitive restructuring specialist named Donalee Markus for a brain injury, and who raved about Markus's effectiveness. The next morning we called Dr. Markus (hereafter "Donalee," as everyone calls her, but intended with the greatest respect and fondness), reached her on her cell phone, and began, in that moment, the transformation that gave me back my life.

---

*It was the fascinating book by Norman Doidge, M.D., *The Brain That Changes Itself: Stories of Personal Triumph from the Frontiers of Brain Science* (Penguin, 2007), that started us looking for those connected with brain plasticity research. Dr. Doidge very graciously wrote back to my inquiry—the only one. He was, understandably, somewhat overwhelmed by the flood of e-mail he was receiving, and did not have any immediate ideas, though he kindly suggested writing to him again if I still was at a dead end. By then we had found Dr. Donalee Markus.

PART THREE
THE GHOST RETURNS

MEET DR. DOTS!

Even in our first, brief phone conversation I found Donalee Markus inspiring. She is one of those people just bursting at the seams with life, and compassion, and goodwill. We traded information and agreed to meet at her home office.

Donalee is a *cognitive restructuring specialist* who practices clinically applied neuroscience—meaning that she reconfigures people's brains so that they see the world, and think, differently. To achieve her ends she has developed specialized visual puzzles that change the low-level building blocks of thought itself. She has treated hundreds of people over a thirty-year career—many of whom, like me, have suffered traumatic brain injuries. She has led seminars on maximizing intelligence for prestigious institutions like NASA and Los Alamos National Laboratory, written books, appeared on television many times, and developed online intelligence-boosting puzzles.

Although Donalee is now past the age when many have already retired, she still rises by five every morning to get to work, and appears to have the energy of a woman in her twenties. The word "dynamo" comes to mind when you meet her in person. One can't help but be charmed.

On January 31st, 2008—more than eight years after the crash—I met with Donalee at the beautiful Highland Park home she shares with her surgeon husband. We went downstairs into her basement office, and I sat across a table from her as we talked. We were surrounded by cheerful colors and interesting objects, including attractive candy bins—an indication of her work with children—and also a large number of file cabinets and drawers filled with many thousands of different cognitive puzzles. Donalee and I discussed a partial list of my symptoms, and also a list of my cognitive/personality weaknesses and strengths prior to the crash, both of which she had asked me to prepare in advance. I explained the difficulties I was having, and that I had more or less reached the end of the line, despite my best efforts to the contrary. To my surprise, she understood immediately about the unworkable cognitive load from my inability to filter out Erin's constant chatter.

After some preliminaries during which I made drawings with colored markers, Donalee had me sit at a table and make a copy of the line-drawn design shown in Figure 3.

Looking at the drawing, I told Donalee that I knew exactly what was going to happen, and that within a few minutes I would be rather affected by the effort of what she was asking of me—even though ordinarily it would be trivial to make a copy of so simple a figure. She wanted to see how I approached the

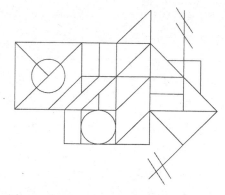

Figure 3: Complex Geometric Line Drawing

task anyway, as this was one of her diagnostic tools. So I set about copying the abstract drawing onto a blank piece of paper.

Within a minute I began to lose normal control of my muscles; my hands and upper body grew contorted. Over the course of the next five minutes, my symptoms steadily worsened. My eyes grew wide like saucers. I hunched over the paper with my head twisted sideways, about six inches from the table. I looked very much like a person having a neurological meltdown—like an outwardly normal Professor Jekyll transforming before everyone's eyes into a bizarre Mr. Hyde with cerebral palsy. I stared intensely at minute pieces of the design, trying to make sense of them, to "see" them, so that I could make the transfer to the new page. I worked ever more slowly . . . slowly . . . slowly . . . methodically copying the simple lines and circles, and finally moving at the speed of a frame-by-frame slow-motion movie. My movements became increasingly uncoordinated as the muscles in my arms, neck, face, back, and hips knotted up. The paper got bunched and wrinkled as my left hand, holding it, became increasingly contorted. While completing the task I kept up a calm, joking dialogue in slightly slurred speech, saying things like, "Well, as I said, this always happens. I try to avoid this kind of activity if I can help it."

Donalee told me later that in watching me work she was stunned. She had never seen anything like it. Her assistant, Mara, who was in the room, was on the verge of calling 911—giving hand signals to Donalee behind my back asking what to do. Only my calm, oddly juxtaposed, ongoing narrative convinced them to wait and see.

Despite the persistence of my symptoms, Donalee next gave me some simpler tests, and we talked. She had me try on various colored sunglasses: purple, magenta, aqua, and so on.* Surprisingly, the aqua and purple glasses seemed to help my neurological symptoms—my coordination and balance improved, recovering slightly from the breakdown caused by the stress of her tests—and she gave me a pair of each to take home.

In those first two hours we spent working together, I found Donalee to be really engaging—smart, organized, and compassionate. Her knowledge of clinically applied neurology was vast. I could tell that she "got it" right from the start. And critically important to understanding how she works is that she *pays close attention* to the people with whom she works. She is watching, and thinking, and asking, and listening—teasing out small clues to what is going on in the brain.

Donalee told me she would think about what she had observed. I thanked her, and headed out.

As I left, Donalee was again taken aback at the difficulty I had making it through the doorway of her office. She didn't

---

*These can be cheaply purchased. Search for "Color Therapy Glasses" on eBay, though I recommend a healthy skepticism when reading the various therapeutic claims, which have nothing to do with Donalee's application.

know quite what to make of the weird gyrations I used to get my body up the stairs to the first floor: holding on to the wall, twisting my head around and tipping it sideways in odd ways, staring intently at tiny pieces of the visual landscape, raising my arms up as though to fend off an attack from the ceiling and walls as I tried to "see" them in some elemental, proprioceptive way. She was amazed at the deterioration that had taken place just from the simple diagnostic exercises she had given me. I assured her that it was nothing to worry about—that this was normal and I had everything under control.

After I left, I felt quite unsettled. I had been to many doctors and the result was always the same: they never called back. When I went to see them, they had little to offer. I knew this, but once again had allowed myself just a little hope. And yet I saw that, after all, I was once again just going to have to face the fact that my life as I had known it—now almost a decade ago—was well and truly over.

It was embarrassing to be at Donalee's and let on about the extent of my cognitive impairments, and it was saddening to be reminded of how even the simplest cognitive tasks were almost impossible for me to manage. Despite Donalee's obvious compassion, I felt like the humiliation of my life had just been rubbed in my face once again. It evoked unpleasant memories of the time I had gone to see the movie *Memento*. A new low, after all.

Erin, now three, was on a rare visit to the babysitter. So, instead of going home, I took a detour and went to the movies again. I spent several hours there just watching the scenes go by, drifting from theater to theater, not really able to understand what the movies were about, but letting the music, the dialogue, and the visual scenes wash over me in a multisensory montage.

In the late afternoon I went home. Just as I got up to my bedroom to rest for a few minutes before going to get Erin, the phone rang. It was Donalee. *She had called me back.* I couldn't believe it.

Donalee: "Where have you been? I've been trying to reach you all afternoon."

Clark: "I'm sorry. I was upset about having you see me like that. So I went to the movies."

Donalee: "Clark, I have some ideas about how we can approach this. I have a plan. We can deal with this. I don't like to sit around. I want to get this done."

Clark: "What!?" (I was at a loss for words—I couldn't make sense of it.) "I don't know what to say . . . I don't understand."

Donalee: "Why not? What are you talking about?"

Clark: "I've been to see lots of medical people over the last eight years. Once they get a look at me, no one has *ever* called me back."

Donalee (brushing off my amazement): "Well, I'm different, and I know how to work on this problem. One thing I was trying to figure out was, how can you possibly work at all? I've seen how you are. I know exactly what's going on in your brain. There's no way you can work with that kind of brain damage—especially as a professor."

Clark: "To be honest, it hasn't been very easy."

Donalee: "Then I realized what it is. *You're the guy that never gives up—ever!* Right?"

Clark (pausing, thinking): "Hmm. Well, yes. That's who I am."

Donalee (humorously): "Ever! . . . Ever!! . . . EVER!!!"

We both laughed.

Donalee: "I can work with that. We can fix this, Clark. I know where to start, and we'll take it from there. When can you come back to see me?"

And Dr. Donalee Markus was right. She *did* know what to do. This was the beginning of the brain-plasticity miracle that gave me back my life, and that we'll now see unfold *before my eyes.*

BRAIN GLASSES

Part of Donalee's plan was that I also work with a colleague of hers, Deborah Zelinsky, an optometrist who emphasizes neuro-optometric rehabilitation. Donalee's comment was "We can manage everything here at my office, but in your case it will probably go faster if you also work with Debbie. Go visit her and see what she says."

So the following week I went to see Deborah Zelinsky, O.D., F.N.O.R.A., F.C.O.V.D.,* for the first time. Dr. Zelinsky (hereafter just "Zelinsky" as she seems often to be referred to, out of respect for her uniqueness, like "Bach" or "Einstein") is a brilliantly innovative neuroscientist in a clinician's white coat. She

*Optometry Doctor; Fellow, Neuro-Optometric Rehabilitation Association; Fellow, College of Visual Development.

accesses the brain primarily through manipulating the light that passes through our retinas. Coming from an academic family that includes a former Northwestern University professor of mathematics, and a Caldecott Medal winner, Zelinsky regularly engages in scholarly activities such as giving seminars on her techniques in many European countries, attending scientific sessions, and occasionally chairing them. She was the 2013 recipient of the Neuro-Optometric Rehabilitation Association Founding Fathers Award—a distinction she shares with the eminent scholar V. S. Ramachandran, who received the award in 1997. She has worked with the blind, the autistic, the developmentally delayed, those who have had traumatic brain injuries, children with learning problems, and other special populations. She serves as an expert witness for brain-injury cases.

Zelinsky maintains a suburban practice north of Chicago called *The Mind-Eye Connection* and between lectures that take her around the world sees patients as an optometrist who makes use of many neurodevelopmental rehabilitation techniques. Although she is a talented and practicing optometrist, and regularly prescribes glasses for patients, it is clear after spending just a few minutes with her that she is primarily focused on how the visual systems interact with brain function, and how the visual/spatial functions in the brain are integrated with the higher-order brain processing that makes us human.

When I first entered the Mind-Eye Connection offices, the immediate thought that came to mind was *friendly commotion*. Zelinsky's office, and lab, is the informal hub of not only a local, but also a national and even an international network of people wandering through one of the great, casual unfoldings in clinical brain science. On this visit there was a local high-school student sitting in the waiting area, there for a pair of glasses; a developmentally challenged third grader from Ohio trying on frames in the display foyer; and a European neuroscience professor wandering out from one of the examination rooms where he had been chatting with a pair of top-notch optometry interns from California.

On the front desk there was a pair of glasses that needed a screw replaced, sitting next to some notes for a presentation on her work that Zelinsky was giving the following week. The receptionist was talking on the phone to a parent from Texas who was desperately trying to slip her child into Zelinsky's packed schedule. In the receptionist's free hand was Zelinsky's travel packet for yet another series of lectures she'd be giving in Europe later in the year.

Zelinsky herself came out of a different examination room holding a patient's folder, momentarily resumed the ongoing academic conversation she'd been having with the neuroscientist, then stopped to give a charming smile to the third grader—complimenting the little girl on her choice of frames. Zelinsky introduced herself to me, then handed me off to her assistant Martha.

In all I spent three hours that day in testing and diagnostic interviews, interleaved with the other patients—first with Martha, and then with Zelinsky herself.* The later parts of the testing were conducted in Zelinsky's examination room, using her phoropter (the lens-swapping optometric machine that fits over a patient's face). Zelinsky took copious notes throughout the process, and often referred back to earlier test results as she tried different combinations of lenses.

---

*It is typical that an initial appointment with an optometrist emphasizing neuro-optometric rehabilitation will take one and a half to three hours because of the extensive testing needed.

Zelinsky explained that she would prescribe for me a special pair of glasses that included, among other things, prisms. They would not correct my eyesight the same way my regular glasses would, and they would not be useful for reading. She cautioned me about driving with them on. Beyond that, she wanted me to wear them as much as I could tolerate—it would take work on my part because the glasses were going to push my brain in the direction she wanted to take it. "Change is not always easy," she said.

I had brought with me extensive notes on my symptoms, which I was prepared to discuss with Zelinsky. At Donalee's urging, I particularly wanted to go over with her the "visual brain seizures" that caused my body to contort and my limbs to shake from side to side under certain kinds of brain stress. Zelinsky was not the least bit impatient with me, but was understandably anxious to move on to the other appointments she had queued up. "I read through everything you brought me while you were working with Martha," she explained. "We don't need to discuss your notes. I already know what's wrong with you." I was a little taken aback. "And I know how to fix it," she added, before giving me a quick nod and a smile, and then walking away to greet her next patient.

And indeed, she did know how to fix it.

A few days later I got my first pair of "brain glasses"—my *Phase I* glasses, as I later came to call them. In the days that followed, my cognitive functioning improved dramatically—no, let's say astoundingly—and for the first time in eight years I started to feel like a real human. The effect of the new glasses, along with the work I had started pursuing with Donalee, was stunning. Importantly, although it was tiring and challenging for me to make the transition, it also felt *right*.

Within the context of Donalee's simultaneous treatment, Zelinsky was able to achieve, for the price of an office visit and a pair of glasses—and within the course of ten short days—what some of the leading neurologists in Chicago, and a famous rehabilitation center, and many others, had claimed would never happen: I started to get better.

While I was understandably blown away by the dramatic results, Zelinsky was mostly cavalier about it. She was, of course, happy that I was getting better, but she already knew what would happen because she had seen it many times before. She knew what she was doing. This was old hat for her.

I've preserved a letter I sent to Zelinsky just two weeks after getting my first pair of glasses, and in looking at excerpts from it we have a window onto this remarkable period during which my brain was starting to reconfigure itself.

Clark Elliott
[. . .]
Evanston, IL

28 February 2008

"The Music Behind My Eyes"

Dear Dr. Zelinsky,

Below are some further notes that fall into the "very strange" category. [. . .] I thought it best not to mention these current symptoms when I saw you in person because, well, they are just odd, and there wasn't time to explain.

However, since you were trying various glasses on me *with my eyes closed* on Tuesday (!), and since we did briefly discuss the "blindsight" phenomenon involving non-visual retinal processing, it seems that I might best give you this additional data. I suppose I am trusting that you will not think me to be a mental case.

There are two (additional) not-at-all subtle alterations that coincide with my having worn the glasses for about ten days. However, they both have to do with my *hearing*.

First, some background: Before becoming a professor of Artificial Intelligence I attended the Eastman School of Music, and also spent time studying conducting, and trumpet, as a part-time student at the Juilliard School. I was one of the least naturally-talented *musicians* at either school. However, I was known as having one of the truly exceptional ears for "sound," such that many recitalists would bring me in before concerts to tweak the hall, sound stage, and so on.

I left music school to have more time to devote to my musical ear. To this end, I spent more than a year listening to single notes, then gradually two, and then three, on the piano, roughly eight hours a day, studying their individual sounds, and developing my ear. I have continued to study music, and in particular musical *sound*, listening pretty much every day for the last thirty years, with a few years' forced hiatus after my brain injury.

Now fast forward to last week.

Strange Point One:

I typically listen to music with my eyes closed, and last week I began to notice something odd happening. With my glasses off (note: with my eyes CLOSED) I would hear the sound coming from my stereo speakers (which were fourteen feet away) contained within the borders of an imaginary approximately 50 degree angle starting just behind my eyes and reaching toward infinity past the speakers. This was "normal."

But, with the new glasses on (and my eyes closed), the sound stage instantaneously came about "ten feet" closer,* and, most dramatically, the angle of my "hearing-scape" changed to 180 degrees, extending in a straight line through just behind my eyes, and encompassing everything in front of that line.

For someone with ears as acute as mine, this is not a subtle difference.

What do I mean by my hearing being *different*? Well, this is a little hard to describe. I suppose I have always known that I "see" sounds. That is, I hear them, but I represent them as visual symbols. Sort of like: when listening intently I am not using my eyes at all, but I am hearing the sounds visually through my ears.

With the glasses on I have more than tripled the space in which I process the meaning of sound. But, it is much more profound than a face-value "3x" increase. For example, when I study music I use every available piece of *working memory* to store what I'll call "partial products of my listening process." When this temporary, ephemeral space in which I can "see" and "hold" my hearing increases three-fold, I get an orders-of-magnitude increase in the complexity of sound that I can process.

Overall, the result is that there is an important and

---

*That is, it was as though I were actually sitting ten feet closer to the performers, with the sound tending to wrap around me, instead of being in front of me.

dramatic qualitative increase in the depth of my listening, rather than a quantitative one.

The 180 degrees of my hearing (a 130 degree increase) applies primarily horizontally, but also, to a lesser degree, vertically.

Strange Point Two:

One point of immediate understanding with other people I have met who also have had serious TBI is that we understand one another when we say, "I am no longer human." That is, in my case, I am sort of like a human, and I can fake it such that no one else notices, but something very tangible is missing. I imagine it to be like having had some kind of mystery lobotomy.

Starting around the middle of last week I started noticing an improvement with this problem. An old friend, like the ghost of who I used to be—the real me—started following me around.

Although I cannot describe why this is so, "that" me seems strongly connected to my "180 degree hearing." That is, he had to go somewhere else because he could not live in the impoverished representational soundscape that I was able to support. But now, at least temporarily, and from time to time, I've had enough hearing space to get a glimpse of the old me.

We are listening, profoundly, through our magic internal eyes, to the rich world around us.

Best regards,

Clark

THE GHOST

In fact, in the letter I was holding back. My fear was that Ze-linsky would think I was out of my mind—a nutcase. I thought it best to give her the data, but I was also hesitant to say too much.

Here are more details:

The difference in my hearing was *remarkable*.

I am a serious "audiophile" in that I treat my stereo system as though it were a fine musical instrument. Over the course of twenty years I worked with a reclusive genius to build it with special silver wire, vacuum tubes manufactured in England in the late 1950s, and resistors and capacitors from specialty suppliers all over the world. I listen through homemade speakers that have been built and rebuilt dozens of times as I chased a particular sound. I listen to music coming through my stereo as one might listen to Brahms coming through a Stradivarius violin.

When my stereo system is "locked in," all thought of the equipment evaporates. It is impossible to focus on anything but the musical performance being reproduced. This is how one knows the system is *right*. And I have never been able to stand the harsh, rhythmless, flat sound that comes from compact discs, so I listen only to vinyl—records.

One evening, a week after getting my glasses, I found some time in my schedule to sit down and listen to music. I put on a record, sat in my listening chair, closed my eyes, and let the sound wash over me.

Within the first few bars of the music I was so startled that I leapt up out of my chair, wondering what was going on. I know my stereo system inside out. I know my recordings inside out. I listen so carefully, so attentively to the details of the sound, that even a minor change becomes apparent. But I certainly was not familiar with the sound I was now hearing! It had been years since I had heard anything so . . . *coherent*. I couldn't believe it. I wondered if perhaps there was some major change in the quality of the electrical power coming from ComEd, which can affect stability in the musical sound. I checked over my equipment, and everything was the same as always.

So I sat down again, and closed my eyes, and thoroughly, gratefully—blissfully—enjoyed the music. I could not believe how cohesive it was, how much complexity I could make out in the visual/spatial, symbolic internal vision I always projected in my mind's eye to make sense of the relationships I heard in the music. I could feel, and "see," the pull—the *stretching*—in the rhythm of the bass in a way that perfectly offset the downward leaping steps of the melody, and with a haunting open har-mony set off in the inner voices.

At one point, still with my eyes closed, I took my glasses off so I could better relax and just enjoy the music—and the vision immediately disappeared! Instantly, I could no longer hear the magic in the sound. The musical *vision* became in-stead only a haunting memory. I was on the outside looking in, through opaque glass.

So I put the glasses back on, with my eyes closed. And . . . once again I could "hear" my internal, almost ethereal, vision of the music. This was dumbfounding. My scientific curiosity was piqued: how could wearing glasses so drastically change my *hearing*, especially *with my eyes closed*?

With the glasses on, my brain systems converged into a kind of "focus" that allowed for a much broader internal visual canvas on which I could arrange the symbols of my thinking. When I put on my new glasses, the immediate result was that, at least in some ways, my effective working memory expanded, or perhaps my access to it did. This allowed for many times the complexity in my cognitive reasoning. I had much more room in which to work: I could use the entire 180-degree space around my head, to the sides and front, for visualizing the music.

By the second week of wearing my new glasses I had the strongest feeling that someone was following me around. At first, whoever it was, was lurking about twenty feet back, and a few feet to the right, off my right shoulder. Each day this person—or thing, or presence, or apparition, or ghostly presence—got a lit-tle closer, but was always behind me, and always behind my right shoulder. If I turned around, *the Ghost* moved around too, so that it was still behind me. If I twisted my head over my right shoulder to get a look at it, it would dart just beyond the periphery of my vision.

Although I could never see who it was, I had the strange "sense" that this entity was about as tall as I was. It wasn't so much that I was in contact with a sentient being, but was more a distinct change in the way I "felt" the world, or heard it, in that particular area of the three-dimensional space around me.

This was spooky, and I have to admit that I wondered if I was finally losing it, crossing over into the territory of being not just cognitively impaired, but also, maybe, a little nuts. Was this, possibly, the beginning of something really serious, like schizophrenia?

But at the same time that this definitely odd experience was unfolding, I also had a sense of well-being, a feeling that it was all right to let down my constant vigilance. I got used to having the presence follow me around, and it became almost like a companion, sort of like Conrad's *secret sharer*—only mute.

During this whole period, if I was awake, I felt the presence. Each day it came closer, and even during a single day it came closer, inching slowly toward me as it followed me around.

Except for the strange feeling of this apparition, I was in most other ways getting noticeably better. My thinking was clearer. I no longer had to hold on to walls to walk down a corridor. I could think for short periods without nausea. I was able to get the key into my office door, even after teaching—something I'd not been well able to manage for years. I could mostly follow, in real time, what people were saying to me.

After class one evening, I was walking back along the hallway to my office. The Ghost had gotten really close by this time—it was only a few feet away, still behind me, still off my right shoulder.

All at once I realized what was happening: The ghostly presence was *me*. It was the me with whom I had memories back to the time I was three years old watching a toy cement mixer sitting in the sunlight on a windowsill, using that sunbeam to form my first concept of angles. It was the me that had ridden his bicycle up to the University of California to study math and physics when he was eleven years old. It was the me that had so loved his students as he taught music for years, and gone to Eastman, and the me that had finished a Ph.D. while raising his young children and working full-time. It was the me that, so importantly, could deeply, passionately feel the interweaving intricacies of music. It was the me that could talk to God. It was the me that could *think*, and *feel*.

I was overcome with emotion. I always liked that guy, and now, after eight years of exile, he was, at last, coming home. I went into my office and just marveled at what was happening. I was so excited that I was trembling, and grinning uncontrollably from ear to ear, while tears of pure unchecked joy fell on my desk.

By the next day *the Ghost* had moved inside me, from behind my right shoulder. I was, after all this time, reintegrating with myself. At last I had enough brain power to support the real me, the complex me. I could see the world through my own eyes again, could hear it through my own ears, and could apprehend the meaning of the world around me through the prism of my own personality. I was, at last, and once again, *human*!

PART FOUR
THE SCIENCE OF BRAIN PLASTICITY

How had this happened?

Everything had occurred so fast that I couldn't make sense of it. I had had no time to adapt. It was like blinking and then waking up from an eight-year dream—still less than a month since Heather had even heard of Donalee Markus in the first place. I was amazed that these treatments *worked*. In all the time since the accident, *nothing* I'd tried had made the slightest bit of difference. Now I put on "magic glasses" and did connect-the-dots puzzles, and within two weeks I was suddenly getting better.

Before meeting with Donalee and Zelinsky, I hadn't made any effort to research the scientific techniques behind what was now, for me, a miracle. But as the fog lifted and I started to return to a semblance of normal life, my professor's curiosity started nagging at me. Why did *these* treatments work, where all else had failed?

Over the course of the next six months I would continue to improve. During that time I would work hard on the demanding tasks that Donalee set for me to master, and I would also during this period move on to my Phase II and Phase III glasses from Zelinsky, followed in the years after by Phases IV, V, and VI. Although the most significant part of my return to health had now come in the first few weeks of treatment, I still had a ways to go.

To make sense of the process we must look in detail at the remarkable science behind my brain's recovery, starting in those first few weeks and extending through the years that followed. We'll put on our lab coats and our sleuthing hats, looking carefully at what cognitive restructuring specialists and optometrists emphasizing neurodevelopmental rehabilitation do, and also at the details of my own experience in going through the process.

DONALEE MARKUS AND HER DESIGNS FOR STRONG MINDS

"I want to get you in and get you out," Donalee said at our second meeting. "I'll talk with you along the way, but I am not interested in any kind of 'talk therapy.' We'll focus strictly on restructuring the cognitive aspects of your brain, based on neuroscientific principles. My research and training are strictly as a cognitive psychologist, not a clinical one.

"I'll be giving you a series of exercises designed to restore basic cognitive functioning that was damaged in the accident. We'll be working from the ground up. When you've mastered the easier exercises, we'll move on to the next level."

At the time, I was again in her basement office, surrounded by the ubiquitous file drawers full of puzzles. We were starting on the plan she had laid out for my recovery.

"We need to go over your background," she went on, "looking

for lifelong weakness in cognition, such as organizational problems, trouble following rules, or maybe difficulties in integrating the big picture with the detailed view. Such prior weaknesses are the areas most likely to be affected by TBI in a pronounced way."

It was of interest to Donalee that there had been long-undiagnosed, but quite pronounced, attention deficit disorder (ADD) in my family, and although I had always managed this aspect of my life well, I, too, had at least a tendency toward attention difficulties. Donalee used this, along with other information from her testing, to tailor the exercises she gave me.

"There are also strengths to consider," she said. "Like many of the people I work with, you are a very high-functioning individual, and you also, additionally, have a prestigious Ph.D. This becomes very important when we set a baseline for our work together. 'Normal' functioning for you won't be 'normal' for someone else. So the work has to be adjusted."

Donalee now pulled out a drawing I had completed for her thirty minutes earlier and put it on the table between us. When I had first arrived, she'd given me this drawing—similar to the one that had caused me so much trouble on my first visit (see Figure 3, page 207)—but this time she'd had me use a series of colored markers for the task. The exercise had been timed, and after I had copied for a while using one color, she would have me discard that marker and use a new color, in a prescribed order. This way we could see not only the results of my work, but also the *way* in which I had gone about the task.

"We have to take into consideration your general cognitive makeup," she said. "What is your thinking style?" She pointed to the large shapes I had copied with the first colored marker. "In your case we can see that you started out by focusing on these large geometric shapes, then you connected them to form the big picture—the outline—and lastly, you filled in the details. You tend to see problems like this immediately as collections of concepts. Others will focus on the details first and just start copying everything in one small area. There is a wide range of styles that tend to follow professions and also personalities. Managers, for example, will often focus first on the big picture, and have little interest in the details.

"I consider you, and my other clients, as *students*," she explained. "We are going to be teaching your brain *how to learn* again, starting with the cognitive basics.

"We'll be working at a number of different levels," she went on. "For example, in your case it's critical that we repair the connections to the visual cortex that I can see have been damaged in the car accident. We might also have exercises to make sure that your inner *metadialogue*—the ongoing thought-dialogue that distinguishes us from other animals—is working at the appropriate level. Because of your prior tendencies toward attention problems, we're going to work at teasing out what cognitive rules apply in novel situations, and when. Then we'll have you learn to follow them appropriately, step by step."

She asked me questions—teasing out my comfort level—as I worked through a series of various sample puzzles that she took out of the file drawers. She observed me very closely, noting the orientation of my eyes, my motor coordination, and the choices I made. Finally, having tweaked her plan, she gave me a large stack of papers containing puzzles and other exercises to work on, and I left with careful instructions about how to proceed until I saw her again.

"I'm on this, Clark. We're going to fix this!" she said as I left.

I saw Donalee regularly, every two weeks, until June 2008. In all, I visited her nine times over those first six months, and then once again for a follow-up a year later. I had daily homework assignments, which I collected and brought back for her to look over each time I returned.

During these "brain lessons" with Donalee, I went through reams of exercises printed out in stapled collections of sheets, always working with a pencil. And I worked at them virtually every day, limited only by the requirement that I be able to function in other areas of my life after my brain grew tired from doing the exercises.

The practice was always the same: pay attention to the instructions and the training examples, work toward the intended goal, rehearse the exercises over and over again. *Attention, Intention, Rehearsal:* Donalee's mantra. The exercises started out simple, and then, as the earlier tasks were achieved, got increasingly more difficult. I followed a scaffolding model that was based on—and assumed mastery of—the earlier exercises.

"I'm giving you *experiences* in the form of these pencil-and-paper exercises," Donalee told me during one of my visits, "but also *techniques* for solving problems. Presumably these latter will be internalized through your extensive practice of the puzzles, and you'll be able to generalize them to other cognitive problems that arise."

Donalee tailored my specific exercises carefully each week. She was always ready with some new tweak for the plan. I wondered—how many times had she been through this before?

"I've worked with possibly fifty students like you over the years—people with identified traumatic brain injuries," said Donalee thoughtfully. "I've had hundreds of others that have come to me with all sorts of brain problems, the roots of which aren't known."

"I'm wondering . . ." I said. "A number of my students at DePaul show up with one sort of learning problem or another. In talking with the students I've often questioned whether some of these problems are the result of a long-forgotten, or undiagnosed, concussion earlier in their lives."

"We always have to suspect that might be the case," said Donalee.

THE GEOMETRY OF COGNITION. In my work with Donalee, I began by viewing pages of line-drawn two-dimensional shapes, like triangles, squares, and trapezoids, which had dots in the corners. Then, on the subsequent pages, looking at only the dots, or dots with some lines, I started filling in the missing line segments in the drawings to restore the original design (see Figure 4, below).

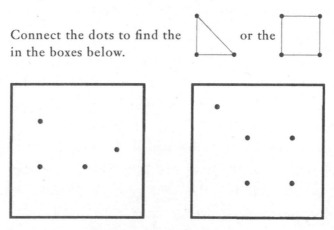

Figure 4: Simple Dots Figures

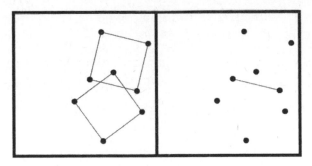

Figure 5: Simple Figures Overlaying One Another

These exercises started very simply, but then got increasingly more difficult as the shapes began to overlay one another, with more of them per exercise, and fewer clues to distinguish the shapes hidden in the dots (see Figure 5, above). Donalee explained our work this way: "You've been trying to run a marathon with a broken leg—your brain—for these last eight years. It can't heal that way. We'll get there, but first we have to go through a step-by-step healing process. In the first of these dots exercises it's like you're lying in the hospital with a cast on, and we're teaching you to wiggle your toes. Once you can wiggle your toes without pain, we'll think about having you sit up in bed. Crutches are a long way off!"

After a couple of months, I graduated to pages and pages of three-dimensional dot exercises. I was first shown the 3D shapes, then given exercises to complete based on those shapes (see Figure 6, page 233).

The first of these exercises had all the dots, and most of the lines, but some of the lines (the "edges" of the shapes) were missing. The exercises then got gradually harder until the lines disappeared altogether, leaving only the dots.

Over time I began to work with arrows, diamonds,

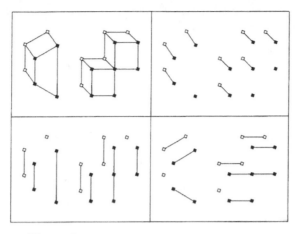

Figure 6: Snippet of 3D Figures with Helper Lines

pyramids, rectangular boxes, octagon-shaped bass drums, and so on. In each case, a shape first appeared on a page by itself. Then different shapes began to appear together. Then they appeared together and were also overlapping. There were page after page after page of dots that had to be connected. By the end, I was given full pages of chaotic-looking sets of dots. All of the 2D and 3D shapes had to be teased out, and drawn with pencil, such that all of the shapes were correctly constructed from connecting the right dots and all of the dots were used (see Figures 7 and 8, page 234 and 235; two full-size dots puzzles appear in the appendix, pages 299 and 300, for readers who want to try them out).

When I brought my homework back to Donalee, she carefully went over every page, every shape, looking for the slightest deviation that would give her clues to my brain state, brain weaknesses, my intentionality about doing the homework, how the motor coordination in my hands was working, and so on.

After a while, we simultaneously began practicing rules

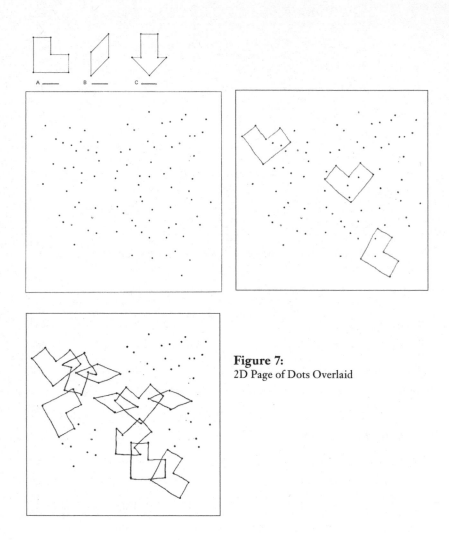

Figure 7:
2D Page of Dots Overlaid

that applied to collections of simple colored objects like balloons and butterflies. The rule might be "find the object that DOES NOT belong in this set." Then I would have to *exactly* follow those rules to complete the subsequent exercises.

For example, in Figure 9, page 235, have we circled all of—and only—the figures that are the *same color*, but *different shape*, from the sample in the square box? (No, because the colored butterfly is not white, the colored lock is neither the same color nor a different

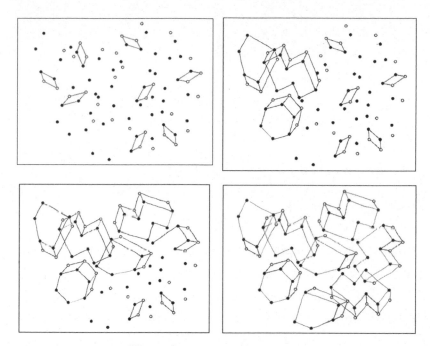

Figure 8: 3D Page of Dots Overlaid

shape, and the white lock is not a different shape, so none of them should be circled; the lower right white butterfly meets the constraints but is not circled.)*

In the early exercises I was given explicit in-

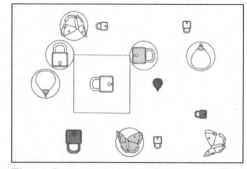

Figure 9:
Snippet of Butterflies Locks Balloons Rules

structions. After a while I graduated to working out my own rules

---

*In the original, the colors blue, red, and yellow are used for shading, and there are many more items.

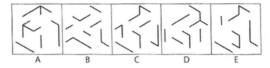

Fill in the blank. Complete the "equations" by
selecting the best answers from the choices below.

Figure 10: Geometric Figure Equations

based on what was implied in an example, and then following those rules to put the objects into correct sets.

I also worked on making perfect copies of many 8.5 × 11 abstract line-drawn schematic pictures that contained parallel line segments, diagonals, circles, triangles, such as the one in Figure 3, and many other types of puzzles.

A difficult kind of geometry puzzle involved creating equations by adding and subtracting one figure from another (see Figure 10, above). These equations ultimately got very complex, with multiple operands.

Sometimes I was given overlapping shapes where I had to remove errors by crossing out lines that connected the dots incorrectly (see Figure 11, page 237).

In all cases the exercises were hierarchical and methodical, were designed to address very specific weaknesses, and were used to bring my symbolic cognitive functioning within normal limits for various kinds of basic cognitive skill categories—that is, importantly, *normal for a very high-functioning intellect.*

When I was working on the intense 2D and 3D mental projections like those in Figure 7 and Figure 8 (pages 234 and 235), Donalee wanted me to draw out the shapes, with pencil, as soon

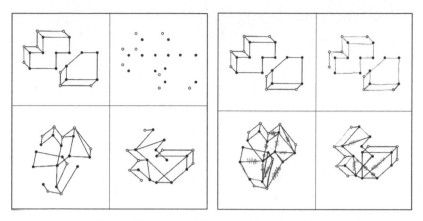

Figure 11: Shapes with Lines in the Wrong Places

as I found them among the cloud of dots. But in keeping with the way I had always studied, I did more than was asked of me. I wanted to get better as fast as possible, and I felt that the harder I worked on these exercises, the sooner I would get back to being myself. So instead of using a pencil, I did the whole of each exercise in my head. I would visualize each of the objects in my mind's eye, and then, keeping that object "alive" (so that I wouldn't accidentally reuse its dots for another shape), I moved on to the next object. In this way I would work through a whole page, often containing fifteen 2D or 3D figures, many of them overlaying one another. At the end I would be able to simultaneously see *all* of the objects rising out of the sea of seventy or more dots as I repeatedly moved from one shape to another in my mind's eye. This gave my eye-aiming systems and cognitive filters lots of guided exercise as I had to repeatedly return to each object to "refresh" the image of it in my mind.*

---

*And as we'll see later, it also reinforced a correct working balance between my central eyesight, which I was using to focus on the object, and my peripheral eyesight, which I was using to set the *context* that allowed me to filter out all the extraneous dots.

Working through a single page of dots the first time might take me forty-five minutes of intense concentration. Because I hadn't actually drawn on the paper—visualizing all the shapes only in my head—I was able to repeat the exercises many times each week. I would then note the number and types of the objects in a coded sequence on the bottom of the page, to later go over with Donalee.

I also took to working through the exercises in a different variation wherein I practiced *as though I were physically drawing the lines*, but without actually picking up a pencil to do so. That is, rather than simply staring at the page waiting for the shapes to "rise out of" the dots, I imagined I could feel my hand holding a pencil, drawing the objects.

I had always been naturally gifted at these kinds of intense symbolic-geometric visualizations as I worked out many kinds of problems, so this was normal mental exercise for me, and was in keeping with Donalee's belief in matching the exercises to baseline cognitive capabilities. I felt that for *my* brain the intensity of doing the many exercises completely in my head was the only way I could ever hope to restore the levels of reasoning I needed for my work as a professor. At times I would concentrate so hard on the exercises that it was as if I were in another world. It was intensely hard work, *but it felt right.*

Yet Donalee was neither mollified nor persuaded. "I need you to actually *write down* your interpretation of the shapes!" she admonished. "I have to check for cognitive deficits in your work, and I need to see how you are drawing your lines. These give me clues about your brain state as you work.

"And look, an important part of the brain's work, as you have seen, is in using cognitive symbols to guide the motor control of your hands, arms, hips, back, and neck muscles. Need

I remind you that you've got a problem there?" She laughed. "We need you to be *physically* translating your inner vision, through your body, into the real world. My exercises are designed to work with these motor skills!"

Despite her objection, we compromised. I would work through the exercises in my own way by visualizing the shapes in my head, and imagining also, in a different version of each exercise, that I was physically drawing them with a pencil. I would do this many times for each exercise, but then, before I returned, I would use a real pencil to actually connect all the dots.

Working through the exercises felt *good*, but despite the great advances I had made, they were still debilitating. After working on them—especially in the first two months—I often could not walk, or do much of anything, so I had to carefully portion out time to work on my homework while leaving enough resources to get through my still-challenging days.

ATTENTION DISORDER AND THE FOLLOWING OF RULES.

"Donalee," I said at one of my visits two months after I had started with her, "I really don't want to be working on these annoying 'find the rule' exercises anymore. I figured them out right away, weeks ago, and they don't present any challenge to me."

The exercises were maddening. Donalee was giving me long collections to work through. I had to flip to a page, read the instructions or tease out the rule, and then, using the instructions or the rule, isolate objects that did not match. It was not in my nature to put much effort into such essentially boring, rote work.

Donalee was adamant. "You have to keep working on them," she replied. "You have a tendency toward attention difficulties.

It runs in your family. In your own case this weakness—which you were able to manage prior to your brain injury—has now become problematic. So it's a brain area we've got to strengthen."

She went on. "In my experience, people with attention difficulties—especially high-functioning people—always find reasons why they shouldn't have to follow the rules. Their reasons take many forms, but often are some subset of 'these rules are stupid and it doesn't make any sense to follow them'—a variation on what you are telling me now.

"In fact, these tactics are mostly, unwittingly, used to mask the problem that attention-disordered people *cannot* follow the rules. They can't attend long enough to do so. Life would often be much easier, less chaotic, and more productive, if they could address their cognitive difficulties such that they could *learn to follow rules.*

"I'm giving you these exercises so that you can identify the rules, and follow them. Just that. Not only do you have to attend to what the rules are, but you have to form the intention to follow them, and then rehearse, over and over again, the following of those rules. Whether you've figured them out, or agree with them, or they suit you, is irrelevant."*

I thought about this and, much to my chagrin, realized that she was right. I came from an intellectually high-functioning, iconoclastic family that generally questioned all rules, and followed them only "when it made sense" to do so. Neither of my parents—each of them a graduate of UC Berkeley—was good at following rules. My parents would happily expend three times

---

*For high-functioning people, this brain weakness is often disguised by the very real problem of spending long hours in school on group tasks that are moving too slowly—a mismatch where anyone would understandably grow restless.

the energy to avoid following a "stupid" rule as it would have taken to simply "waste" the time following it.

"We need to end as much of the chaos in your life as possible," Donalee said bluntly. "It is mentally exhausting for you. You will be needing all of your brain resources to lead a normal life."

Surprisingly, but wonderfully, I found that working through Donalee's puzzles, building solid cognitive capabilities from the ground up, began to translate into real life.

The processes of determining relationships between symbols (such as *part-whole, belongs or doesn't belong, left-to-right ordering, same color/different color*) and of *figuring out the rule, then following it to the letter* were, essentially, the same when manipulating puzzle icons as they were when reasoning about the real world. In both cases the objects and problem-solving procedures got translated into the same internal iconic forms.

Because of all the practice visualizing objects and relationships in the dot puzzles, my ability to generally visualize symbols and relationships from real life gradually got better as well. My ability to figure out the rule in a real-life organizational task, then follow it, got better. My ability to organize visual scenes got better. My ability to balance background context and attentional focus got better. And, the complex 3D puzzles seemed to exercise a very important *spatial* part of my symbolic-reasoning system that I used to solve complex real-world problems.

In particular, my ability to *think* was gradually expanding, and I could do so with less fatigue.

Zelinsky's glasses had given me access to new paths in my brain, and the work with Donalee was pushing my brain to grow and develop along those new channels. The plan made sense. The work made sense. The results were coming.

Thank you, Donalee—you called me back!

DEBORAH ZELINSKY AND THE MIND-EYE CONNECTION

Before we return to Zelinsky's lab to delve into the fascinating world of an optometrist whose work is based on neurodevelopmental research, it's important to first learn something about how the human visual system works. Then we'll walk step-by-step through my recovery using what we have learned to explain the details of *why* treating my brain's visual system was so crucial to my recovery.

A QUICK TOUR THROUGH THE VISUAL SYSTEM. There are three retinal processing pathways through the brain. Two of these, for *central vision* and *peripheral vision*, are for eyesight and are processed in the brain's visual cortex. The third is for *non-image-forming retinal signals* (also primarily from the peripheral part of the retina) that branch off and are processed by other body systems such as for posture control, for sleep rhythms, for the production of melatonin, etc. Each of these is crucial to our well-being, as is the coordination among them.

There are roughly 100 million receptors in the retina of each eye, which respond to light, but there are only a million *axons* leaving the retina, so the many layers of the retina together act as a very sophisticated sensory filter. Additionally, the retina acts as a *transducer* that converts light into neural signals: input *photons of light* enter through the lens, pass through a *chemical stage* in the early retinal layers, and then move on to a later *electrical stage* comprising the neural signals sent out along the axons. Axons are bundled together, depending on which area of the retina they come from, and this also determines the route they will be taking through the brain. The collected bundles of the one million axon output fibers form the *optic nerve* for each eye.

Vision signals spread out and are routed along many different paths known as *optic radiations* to the back of the brain where the visual cortex resides. Different parts of the visual cortex process, first, *movement, location, size, and shape* from the peripheral vision, and, second, lagging just slightly behind, *colors and details* from the center vision (though see the footnote on page 246). This is what is classically thought of as the "visual system."

Thus we have a chain of crucial steps in translating light into meaning: how light is transmitted through the clear cornea and lens of the eye, how the various sections of the retina are activated, how the photoreceptor signals are reduced to the axon output, how activation is dispersed among the various axon bundles in the optic nerve, *how the signal is routed to the visual cortex*, and how the signal is passed on by the visual cortex to the rest of the brain, which gives it meaning.

But we are not done. In the past ten years, retinal research has shown that there are many other *non-image-forming pathways* from the retina to various body systems. These channels affect the "homeodynamics" (dynamic self-organization) of the body—through hormones, enzymes, and other mechanisms. For example, there are receptors linked with thyroid function, pupil dilation and constriction, dopamine production, and adrenaline production. Consider that when light cycles change we can experience jet lag, or seasonal affective disorder, and those who are completely blind may have to deal with circadian rhythm challenges because of *non-24-hour sleep-wake disorder.* One can easily understand the powerful effects of this non-image-forming retinal input as follows: imagine that a gigantic spider suddenly crosses into your peripheral field of vision. A jolt of adrenaline will begin flooding your body well before your conscious mind interprets the threat. In fact these non-image-forming retinal signals are always given precedence: the signals travel faster and are processed first; when our bodies are under high stress we often cannot pay attention to what we are seeing with our central-image visual processing.

And for each of these paths, a complex network of feedback signals continually biases the whole system—altering the information that is passed on to the brain.

Ultimately, almost every part of the brain gets involved, because the processing of visual/spatial information is linked to symbolic thought, body sense, motor coordination, memory, balance, hearing, and so on. Along the way to the visual cortex, signals from other sensory systems are integrated, such as those for hearing and proprioception.

Nor can the retinas be considered as simply input devices, because signals also return to the eye in response to cognition and body states (such as emotions), to make significant chemical and electrical changes in the retina, and to control both eye movement and filtering in the retina. For example, a depressed person may have signals returning to the eye shutting down peripheral awareness (shutting out the world), whereas a person with ADD might have signals *emphasizing* peripheral awareness (distracted by everything). In this way, vision is a complex process, closely integrated with the inner workings of the brain. Note that when we are not looking at anything at all, but simply thinking, our eyes will move in very specific ways according to our thoughts. From a scientific standpoint, our eyes really are windows into our souls.

In her practice, Zelinsky alters the input into each of the two eyesight systems, as well as into the non-image-forming retinal systems, makes very sophisticated measurements and observations of the resulting output, and then uses this information to make deductions about the likely nature of the brain processes leading from the former to the latter.

Critical to Zelinsky's work—as we will see shortly—is the idea that by activating different parts of the retina, she can *alter the paths through the optic radiations* that the retina's eyesight signals will take on their way to the visual cortex, and also *the paths of the non-image retinal signals* that branch off from the optic nerve before they get to the optic radiations.

There are three ways that Zelinsky uses light to alter the way the brain operates. First, she can bend the light to *different parts of the retina*, which, ultimately, activates bundles of axons differently. In other words, the same visual/spatial signals are being sent, but they are being filtered differently (in the reduction from 100 million to 1 million in the retinal layers), and are being routed differently (through different bundles of axons). When we consider that 100 million receptors are packed into about a square inch of the retina's surface area, it is obvious that even very small changes in the optics can make a huge difference in which receptors are being activated.

Second, Zelinsky can change the *frequency of the light* by allowing different colors through to the retina. Roughly speaking, when the frequency of the light changes, different frequency-sensitive photopigment chemicals, such as melanopsin (~480 nanometer wavelength sensitivity) and rhodopsin (~500 nanometer sensitivity), cause different photosensitive receptors in the same area of the retina to become activated. Thus, while the light may still be hitting the same part of the retina, different cells become activated, ultimately changing the output signals in the optic nerve.* The science of this process of frequency filtering gives new meaning to the phrase "seeing the world through rose-colored glasses."

Third, Zelinsky can selectively *block signals from reaching the retina* at all through using occlusion filters that simply reduce, or block out, the light to certain parts of the eye.

With change either to the location of where the light strikes the retina, to the frequency of the light striking it, or to the amount of the light striking it, the result is that the signal load is dispersed differently through the pathways in the brain.

This is where the principles of *brain plasticity*—one foundation of modern brain science—come into play. When the brain is damaged, such as from TBI, it is possible that the retinal output signals might be fine, and the visual cortex might even be in

---

*We now know, from contemporary research, that this chromatic response is not just in the cone cells in the center of the eye, but also extends out to the periphery of the retina as well, thus extending the effect of colored filters on brain processing.

good shape, but the pathways between the two, or the areas around the pathways with which the axons interact, are damaged. Signals along the old paths are degraded (think of "picking up static") because of the permanently damaged tissue. By bending the light in the eyes, selectively occluding it, and changing the frequency of the light, Zelinsky is able to avoid the damaged routes along which the visual/spatial signal travels.

To greatly simplify this staggeringly complex system, considering eyesight only, let's imagine that there are only one hundred different paths along which signals travel from the retina to the visual cortex. Now let's imagine a patient with brain damage from TBI for whom twenty of these paths have become permanently damaged. On suspecting this, Zelinsky would try to change the input to the eye so that the eighty remaining paths were emphasized and used more heavily, and the twenty defective paths were avoided, in carrying the same signal to the visual cortex. Think of rerouting traffic from a highway, U.S. 25—which has been damaged—to highways U.S. 40, U.S. 50, and U.S. 60—which are still in good shape. The same traffic is getting through, but it is taking a different route.

Through habituation, when the new pathways through the brain are established, the healthy tissue adapts, and the magic of the brain's plastic nature takes over. Within a very short time the new brain tissue learns its new tasks in conveying the visual/spatial signals to the visual cortex. Because it is healthy, the signal path is once more restored to its full capacity without distortion. And, once the brain learns to process the signals along the new paths, the need for the remedial help in "jump-starting" the new paths may become unnecessary.

This explains why I tried many kinds of brain exercise over the course of eight years, but only experienced distress, and pain, with even the simplest sorts of intellectual tasks: I was simply repeatedly sending signals along the old, well-worn, but now damaged, paths.* And this is why the standard medical response for brain damage is "learn to live with it, because you'll never get better—no one ever does." And yet, within two weeks of getting my first pair of brain glasses, my plastic brain had reconfigured itself, learning to follow healthy pathways through to the visual cortex—and I was vastly, hugely improved. Additionally, although I can't claim it as part of the science, it is my strong intuition that the constant onslaught from bad visual/spatial signals required parts of my brain to simply shut down because the input was too exhausting to process. Once the signals were sorted out, those parts of my brain—used in complex spatial cognition and symbol manipulation—could come out of hibernation.

WORKING WITH AN OPTOMETRIST EMPHASIZING NEURO-DEVELOPMENTAL REHABILITATION. Having laid the foundation, we can now walk through the processes that Zelinsky uses to translate her knowledge of the image-forming and non-image-forming retinal systems into the practical matter of making people's brains function the way they were intended. The first step is determining the current state of a patient's brain, and for this Zelinsky uses an extensive battery of tests, along with intuition based on her years of clinical experience.

In that first trip I took to Zelinsky's office, I went through more than fifteen different visual/neurological testing procedures, some of them formal, and some of them less so—but

---

*Donalee addresses this problem by starting out with the very simplest forms of rudimentary cognition, and working up only very slowly from there—recall the analogy of the broken leg.

still important information for Zelinsky, who was looking for subtle clues to my brain's organization. Many of the tests were repeated in subsequent visits, with Zelinsky looking for checkpoints as she pushed my brain processing in a very specific direction.

After my brief introduction to Zelinsky, I filled out a long set of questionnaires, and also wrote essay responses about my habits and my specific complaints.* Based on my responses, Martha asked me a series of further questions that helped to diagnose my lifestyle, which in turn gave clues about the organization of my brain. I also brought along several pages of notes on my TBI symptoms that Martha read, summarized in my chart, and then passed on to Zelinsky. I later discovered that Zelinsky *always* read everything I brought her.

The first test Martha gave me was called the *Padula Visual Midline Shift* test. I was told to look straight ahead. Then Martha brought a horizontally held chromium steel shaft, like a skewer for a barbecue, from above down toward the ground so that it gradually entered the middle of my visual field.

She said, "Tell me when the shaft is directly in front of your eyes."

She then repeated the movement, but this time from the ground upward. In this way my top-to-bottom *midline* was determined. The exercise was then repeated from left to right, and right to left.

In normals, these stopping positions will be about the same, and the midlines—horizontal and vertical—will intersect at a

---

*It later turned out that the *style* of my handwriting was as important to Zelinsky as were my answers: Did I slant up or down at the ends of lines? Under certain cognitive loads did I change the spacing between my words? What was the relationship between my writing on the left-hand side of the page and my writing on the right-hand side?

crossing point directly in front of a person's eyes. For those of us with TBI or other brain oddities, the midline may be shifted higher or lower than normal, to one side or the other, or both. In other words, the internal 3D spatial world is no longer lined up with the world coming in through the senses.

According to William V. Padula, the designer of the testing mechanism, when a person has a midline shift—associated with the *ambient visual process**—she may have balance and coordination problems, and have trouble making out the details in a visual scene.[†] Without grounding in this non-image-forming and peripheral retinal processing, the world may become broken into isolated parts, such as what happened to me whenever I went shopping: all the items on the shelves are suddenly experienced as a kaleidoscopic nightmare of overwhelming detail without any context in which to sort them out. The central eyesight processes then have to take over, trying to make gestalt sense of the scene—performing tasks for which they were not designed, causing motor responses to become slower and slower. Cognitive confusion and distress can also result.

I tested normal on the Padula midline test. But as we have seen from previous chapters, I experienced every one of these rather startling symptoms—for reasons other than a midline shift—on a regular basis, suggesting that there were other problems to be found with my ambient visual system.

Next, in the *Yoked Prism Walk*, Martha gave me a pair of

---

*Padula's *ambient visual process* can be described as having two parts: First, and fastest, one of the non-image-forming pathways specifically linked to posture mechanisms—*where am I?* Second, and slower, the part we've already referred to as the peripheral vision—*where is it?*

†William V. Padula and Stephanie Argyris, "Post Trauma Vision Syndrome and Visual Midline Shift Syndrome," *NeuroRehabilitation* 6 (1996): 165–71.

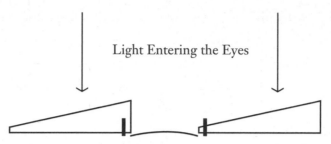

Figure 12: Prism Glasses—Top View with the Yoked Prisms
Shifting Images to the Left

thick prism goggles to wear, and then observed my gait as I walked down the hallway and back four times. Before each trip she adjusted the goggles to a different orientation.

Experientially, prism lenses bend the room in a "fun house" way, tilting it up, sloping it down, and bending the top and bottom in a great arc to the left or to the right, depending on the orientation of the prisms. ("Yoked" means that the prisms are oriented in the same direction.) Although in all cases the visual scene will look altered, patients may have widely differing abilities to walk down the hall from one orientation to another. In my case bending the floor up, and tilting it down, or bending the light from the right, was slightly disorienting, but I was almost immediately able to adjust and navigate the hallway. When the light was bent from my left, though, I became completely disoriented: I had trouble walking and I ran into the side of an open doorway along the way. Such difficulty with one of the lateral orientations is typical for TBI sufferers.

In writing about this test, Zelinsky explains that the Yoked Prism Walk evaluates gross body movements at a reflexive level, as well as spatial orientation, *while the patient is moving*. It can demonstrate how poor stability may impair higher-level perception.*

The distinct discrepancy between my performance with the prisms bending the light left versus bending it right was important—especially when linked to the similar problem I reported, in my notes, of growing dizzy when turning around in one direction, but not the other. This may also have been linked to the phenomenon, discussed earlier, that under brain stress, I was unable to turn to my right at all: I simply could not conceive of "right-ness." And, it may explain other anecdotal aspects of my life as well. For example, if I went running with my daughter, I had to orient *myself* on her left side; when I was on her right, I would start to get dizzy almost immediately.†

Martha next gave me an *Asymmetrical Tonic Neck Reflex* (ATNR) test. "Stand up and hold your arms out in front of you," she said, "like Frankenstein, with your fingers extended . . . Okay. Good. Now turn your head to the left, and then to the right."

ATNR is an innate survival reflex, seen in infants, which often reemerges in adults as a protective mechanism after a shock to the nervous system, such as from TBI. If the subject lowers his opposite arm when turning his head, this suggests a shock has occurred. In my case, an ATNR was present when I turned my head to the left.

---

*Deborah Zelinsky, "Neuro-optometric Diagnosis, Treatment and Rehabilitation Following Traumatic Brain Injuries: A Brief Overview," *Physical Medicine and Rehabilitation Clinics of North America*, Elsevier, 18 (2007): 87–107.

†My notes are clear on this point, that I had to place *myself* on the left-hand side when running and also that I would lose the *right-hand side* of internal visual structures. But because the temporary hemispatial neglect I experienced from time to time was so pervasive when it occurred, I have no *direct* notes at all on being unable to *turn* right; it was not possible for me to take notes on something about which I had no comprehension. I knew only that I had to turn in circles.

Martha then assessed my extraocular muscles—the six muscles that move the eye—using *pursuit tests*, where I tracked the eraser-end of a pencil with my eyes while keeping my head still. She had me follow various patterns, including a big *H*. Martha was looking for any partial paralysis in my eye movements, and also observing my anticipatory eye movements in predicting the path of the target—which gave clues to the peripheral awareness in my brain. Was I able, without thinking about it, to predict the path the eraser was going to take, and adjust my eyes to smoothly follow that predicted path? In my case I had no problem following the pencil, even though, as we saw previously, following a baseball when playing with my boys was extremely fatiguing. The pursuit test results would prove to be important in interpreting the results of later tests.

Martha next gave me a *Near Point of Convergence* test by bringing the pencil close to the bridge of my nose, and then, afterward, the *LANG-STEREOTEST II* to check my stereoscopic vision and depth perception—both of which tested normal.

Lastly, Martha gave me a *King-Devick Test*, in which I read a series of single-digit numbers on two pages. One of the pages just had the numbers on a white background, and the other had lines inserted between one number and the next. The test is used to look for deficiencies in *saccadic eye movements* (extremely rapid, intentional, simultaneous movements of both eyes in the same direction), which can be an indicator of TBI. Tests like this are often used to obtain a quick, objective sideline diagnosis of concussion in football players and other athletes. I tested normal on this exam.

In between completing her work with other patients, Zelinsky would check in with Martha and review some of the

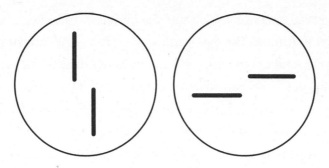

Figure 13: Fixation Disparity Test

data Martha had been collecting. After an hour Zelinsky had me move to her examination room and sit in the phoropter chair, where she began her own testing.

One of the first tests Zelinsky gave me is called the *Super Fixation Disparity Test©*—named after its designer, Dr. Selwyn Super (D.O., F.A.A.O., Ph.D.).* Fixation disparity occurs when the two elements of binocular vision are out of sync.

To get the idea of fixation disparity, consider the circle on the left in Figure 13 above. Note that in the circle there are two vertical line segments—one in the top hemisphere, and one in the bottom. Using occlusions, we arrange it so that each line is seen by only one eye. The measure of misalignment is determined by how far these lines appear to be offset from each other. Testing for disparity is also done horizontally in the same way using the second circle.†

Some alignment disparity is useful as part of the design of the stereo vision system. If monocularly viewed targets are incorrectly misaligned when a person is attempting to view a

---

*Doctor of Optometry, Fellow of the American Academy of Optometry, Doctor of Philosophy.
†Selwin Super, "The Clinical Testing of Fixation Disparity," http://www.professorselwyn super.com/pdf/educator/jbofdarticle.pdf.

scene in the real world, the binocular visual system can usually bring them into alignment and thus avoid double vision. But this is fatiguing, and causes cognitive difficulties—because we are continually refocusing on near and far objects throughout the day, and binocular readjustments have to be made each time. Zelinsky looks to see how much misalignment patients can tolerate in either direction before they lose the ability to synthesize a single stereo image from the two sets of input.

It is believed that in some cases, if such alignment is habitually too far off, the brain will simply shut down the confusing signals from one of the eyes. When this happens it may be true that cognitive functioning in the 3D visual/spatial "internal world" of symbols is also diminished, effectively reducing one's ability to perform complex reasoning and problem solving.

Next, Zelinsky gave me the related *Von Graefe Phoria Test*. Similar to the Super test, Von Graefe measures the habitual tendency of the eyes to point inward, or outward, in the absence of a point on which they can both fixate. Phoria has implications for binocular vision, and the latency period during which the eyes are interpreting binocular visual signals. The test is performed using the phoropter by keeping the image for one eye still, and slowly moving another identical image until the subject reports them as being aligned.

On the Super Fixation Disparity Test©, which takes place in free space (e.g., as per discussion above, all of our "one hundred" imaginary pathways are available from the retina to the visual cortex), Zelinsky found that my overall habitual eye position was slightly outward, though still within the normal range. But on the Von Graefe Phoria Test, which blocks off much of the peripheral vision (so that now only "fifty" pathways are available), she found that my habitual eye aiming was perturbed: my eyes were pointed inward at a distance, and way outward when focused on close-up objects. This caused an exhausting lag in cognition as my eyes had to continually re-aim to avoid double vision. We can imagine the corollary of trying to follow a conversation between two people when, every time we shift our gaze from one person to the other, the audio lags behind the movement of their mouths for a second or two while we struggle to get it to catch up to their gestures.

Next, Zelinsky gave me a *Visual Localization Test*. In this simple (but in my case, ultimately quite telling) test, Zelinsky held a pencil so that the eraser was facing me, about twenty inches in front of my eyes. She said, "Look at the pencil. Then close your eyes and, without looking, reach up and touch it with your fingertip."

She repeated the test with the target in a number of different positions, and also several times specifically had me reach across my body and touch the target with my opposite hand. Despite the theoretical ease of the task, I was completely unable to find the eraser tip of the pencil, with my eyes closed, in any of the positions, helplessly waving my finger around in space until I accidentally hit the target.

In general, a subject's inability to touch the eraser can be caused by three distinct failures. First, the subject may simply not know *where* the eraser is; his central vision allows him to *see* it fine, so he knows *what* it is, but his peripheral vision does not allow him to find it in space relative to his body. Second, the subject might know where the eraser is—his peripheral vision is working fine—but he doesn't know where his hand is. For example, if the subject can reach the eraser on his right-hand side with either arm, but not when the eraser is on his left-hand side, the problem is likely with his visual processing.

If the subject can accurately locate the eraser on either side with one arm, but not the other arm, then the problem is likely with the proprioceptive signals coming from his body. Or, third, in the worst case, he could have problems with both.

In my case, the vision signals going to my visual cortex were fine (eyesight)—this was not the problem. Thus we knew that it had to be the signals coming *from* my muscles, the "where I am" sense, which were not getting through correctly to form an accurate body image in my brain. Zelinsky had two additional clues in interpreting this failure: first, she noted that my severe neck and head pain suggested a compromised motor response sending conflicting signals to my various neck, arm, and back muscles; and second, Martha had noted the ATNR present when I turned my head, indicating that my neck was not operating independently of my shoulders.

Zelinsky followed up with a *Confrontation Visual Field Exam*. She held her hand out to the left side of my head, outside the range of peripheral vision, and said, "Cover your right eye, look straight ahead at my eyes, and tell me when you see my fingers moving." She began wiggling her fingers, at the same time slowly bringing her hand toward the center of my face. As soon as I signaled that I could see her fingers wiggling, she repeated the test on the other side. Zelinsky was determining the volume of space to which I could attend, and was measuring the signals going into my visual system, looking for possible damage to my ganglion cells.

Because I had performed well on the H-pursuit test, successfully anticipating the movement of the pencil through the *H* pattern in the normal way, because my King-Devick Test was normal, and because I demonstrated normal peripheral awareness on the Confrontation Visual Field Exam, Zelinsky knew that the problem was not likely to be with the eyesight system itself.

Lastly, Zelinsky took me through her patented Z-Bell™ Test. The first time one experiences this test, it is quite stunning, and seems almost impossibly magical. While I was sitting in her optometry chair, Zelinsky said, "Close your eyes. When I ring the bell, reach out and touch it with your finger." After my eyes were closed, she brought out a series of differently pitched bells and rang them in various quadrants, high and low, left and right. The test feels *weird* because, with your eyes closed, you can't see anything, so it seems as if you aren't "using" your eyes. And yet, depending on which lenses, tints, and occlusions she uses to alter the light striking your *closed* eyelids, sometimes your hand just waves around helplessly, but at other times you can "feel" exactly where the bell is, and touch it—like feeling the "power of the force" in a *Star Wars* movie.

The key to making sense of this test is in understanding that when the patient's eyelids are closed, no *eyesight images* are registering—he can't *see*—but a significant amount of light is still passing through to the retina. The non-image-forming retinal systems operate with minute levels of light, so they are not affected. In this way we have a quick and easy filter—the eyelids—so we can test the effect of different lenses on the non-image-forming retinal systems, without distraction by the two eyesight systems. We can think of the Z-Bell™ Test as a sort of "vision" test but for non-image-forming retinal processing. This is crucial, because it allows an optometrist to align her patient's three-dimensional *hearing* with his internal visual/spatial map of the surrounding space.

Zelinsky often repeats the test a number of times during

the final phases of tweaking prescriptions for eyeglasses, typically using the phoropter, but sometimes with handheld lenses and filters. Among the treatments she is testing are colored lens filters, prisms, lens prescriptions (possibly including, very specifically, nontraditional balance between the lenses), and translucent occlusions (translucent film applied to the lenses to block, or partially block, light), all later built into the glasses that she prescribes.

The Z-Bell™ Test, already mind-bending to experience yourself, is perhaps equally electrifying to observe. I've now many times watched others being given the test, and what you see is that for one of the bells the patient is waving his finger around eight inches away from where the bell is ringing. He can't find it at all. Then, with just the slightest change in tint, or lens, he is able to touch the bell, right on target, every time.

With no glasses on, and also with my normal prescription glasses for mild nearsightedness, in bright light (and, remember, with my eyes closed), I was not able to touch *any* of the bells in *any* of the quadrants on the Z-Bell™ Test. This was a potential explanation for my great difficulty turning sounds into the visual symbols of thought, and also for my extreme aural sensitivity. Because my visual/spatial system was so degraded, I had to increasingly rely on my audio processing. But, as the Z-Bell™ Tests showed, the 3D spatial world of my hearing was completely out of sync with my 3D visual world, creating an impossibly complex stream of input data that my brain had to disentangle throughout the day. (And we should note that, because of my aural predisposition, and my lifelong study of both sound and music, this integration was much more central to me than it typically would be for others.)

Zelinsky also took me through an exhaustive set of vision tests, such as you might get—in abbreviated form—at a regular optometrist's office ("Which is clearer, A or B?"). Ultimately, she would be prescribing partly for my eyesight, and this had to be taken into consideration, although in my case it was clearly secondary to prescribing for my brain.

Her diagnosis: Except for minor problems with floaters from the crash,* my eyes themselves were working fine. Additionally, the chemical and electrical "magic" that performed the filtering in my retinas was also in good shape, so the reduction from 100 million retinal receptors to 1 million axons was happening correctly. The problem was in my brain. Zelinsky now weighed her options:

1. With the *eyesight* part of any prescription she decided upon, she could affect the relationship between target (center vision, *attention*) and background (peripheral vision, *awareness*). She could blur the target so the background was emphasized, or vice versa. The balance between the two would affect my executive function (i.e., planning and problem solving). She also could make changes in my intentional eye movements, such as where I chose to look within a scene.

2. With *nonyoked prisms*, she could affect my *peripheral awareness* processing, and make changes in my anticipatory eye movements, such as when I was automatically predicting the motion-path of an object.

---

*As a result of the concussion I got floaters (roughly, translucent occlusions in the viscous fluid behind the lens) in both of my eyes. One of my concussion-induced floaters is often situated in the central focus point of my right eye, making it hard to read with that eye.

3. With *yoked prisms*, she could affect my postural mechanisms, and make changes in my orienting movements, such as when I turned my head in response to a sound.

4. Using *filters*, such as tints, occlusions, and the blockage of tear duct drains (tears change the way light gets through to the eye and also help regulate body systems), she could affect the homeodynamics of my body, and make changes in my reflex movements, such as those driven by states of vigilance. For example, there are direct connections between the retina and the hypothalamus, which affects emotion states.

One of the principles of Zelinsky's treatment involves making an additional determination of how much discomfort and challenge a patient can tolerate. Mostly this has to do with the wiring between the eyes and the brain, and is beyond the control of the patient. However, some of it has to do with temperament and how much the patient will work with the lenses to push the brain into using new neural pathways. Often Zelinsky will have to "pry open a small window" in which to work with an early prescription, and then follow up later with a more brain-challenging prescription to get the real work done. With some temperaments, she has found there is not much she can do.

Additionally, any plan Zelinsky formed would, like the plans of Donalee, be both long-term in nature and comprehensive, rather than isolated to a specific condition or problem. In my case, this meant that her plans included fixing processing weaknesses that were present *prior* to my brain injury.

After looking over all the data before her, including my extensive self-reporting notes, Zelinsky made her decisions about treatment. Importantly, she assessed that I could tolerate a lot of discomfort, and also that I was highly motivated to change. She would intentionally push me to the edge of her working window, and would plan on using a series of prescriptions to move me from one phase of brain reconfiguration to the next. I would continue to work with Donalee to exercise my brain and push it to take advantage of its new cognitive capabilities as I progressed with my glasses.

Because I was completely absent the abilities to multitask and plan, Zelinsky felt there were immediate problems to be addressed in my executive functioning. And she also wanted to address serious problems with sensory integration—specifically between my eyes and my ears. She decided that she would work with my "good side," and angle the light from my right (that is, bend the light so that it tended to strike the nasal part of my right eye, and the temporal part of my left eye). For this she used very slight lateral, directive, yoked prisms (0.5 prism diopter in both lenses, with the thick part on the left). But, as noted above, even this very slight prescription was enough to make major changes in which cells of the retina were processing the light. In retesting me on the phoropter, and with hand-held lenses, the Z-Bell™ Test showed me right on target, suggesting that she had found some good pathways through the brain with which to work, and that my eyes and ears were now synchronized.

I was mildly nearsighted, and ordinarily would have been given a slight corrective lens in order to see better. But instead of correcting me to 20/20, Zelinsky wanted to stabilize the background of my eyesight—the peripheral, context-setting vision (in contrast to the central target vision)—so she made the lenses slightly thicker in the center, and thinner on the edges. This scattered the light so that it was dispersed toward the corresponding edges of my retinas, which in turn emphasized my background retinal processing, and deemphasized the target. Zelinsky knew that when I focused on the target I lost my ability to organize the scene surrounding it (such as what happened to me in Home Depot). She wanted me to get more of the context, more of the "bigger picture" of the world around me, and not take in so much of the detail.

This second part of Zelinsky's prescription was intended to address the problems I had when I would become overwhelmed with the details of a visual scene, completely unable to create any gestalt meaning of the larger objects the details comprised: parking lots after shopping, food items on grocery store shelves, and so on. In the diary notes that follow, however, we will also sense my frustration at the necessary (for the moment) diminishing of my central vision.

In the initial days after I began wearing my first pair of glasses I went through all sorts of extreme body and sensory changes, both before and after the Ghost showed up. Having found healthy brain tissue with which to work, I was now relearning how to interpret the signals coming in—like a baby exploring the world. This explains the thrashing that I was going through at the time—waving my arms around in wild gyrations, and dancing, just to walk down a hallway—and the low-level chaos I was experiencing with the apprehension of lines, and doorways, and stairs in my environment. But despite the constant effort, I felt good, and was figuring it all out as my brain rewired itself.

In addition to the phenomenon of the Ghost appearing—which one of Zelinsky's interns suggested might have been partially

caused by some strange form of Charles Bonnet syndrome*—
there were many other odd things happening to me as well. I
took extensive diary notes throughout my treatment with Zelinsky. Following are some entries starting in the first week of
having my Phase I glasses:

> February 8th–25th, 2008: I love the greatly ex-
> panded *hearing* landscape I have with these glasses,
> especially on the left, but I have also considered
> these to be the *glasses from hell!* It is hard for me to
> keep wearing them. They make me so tired, and I
> am always on the border of losing my balance. I
> find myself shouting "I can't see!" (silently, inside,
> but also sometimes even vocally, out of frustra-
> tion) as I try to make sense of the hugely changed
> world around me.
>
> I am constantly hungry, with an incessant crav-
> ing for sugar and carbohydrates. In the very few
> times I have taken the glasses off for an hour or
> so, the hunger recedes. I am gaining weight (two
> pounds a week), but also feel that I am consuming
> many more calories than that.
>
> I am experiencing mild nausea, and mild disori-
> entation much of the time.
>
> I have taken to wearing the glasses twenty-four
> hours a day (that is, I wear them also when I sleep)
> because I have found that with the highly visual

---

*A syndrome in which mentally healthy people—usually with significant visual loss,
and advanced in age—experience purely visual hallucinations, suggested by Grace
Yoon, O.D.

nature of my dreams, without the glasses, I regress by the time morning comes. Wearing the glasses at night allows me to dream without visual fatigue, and I feel much better in the morning.

The glasses have felt "right" (correct) in many profound ways. And yet it is true that, especially early on, at times I have been frustrated to the point of yelling out loud, although even at the time it was happening I couldn't quite describe what it was that was so annoying to me. It was like everything was working correctly, but it was all so new, and I could not make sense of the world around me in the usual way.

This frustration especially tends to happen when I am trying to perform some detailed task like threading a needle, or a cognitive-visual task like finding a particular record album. I have to be careful about knocking things off counters, have trouble getting through doorways and down stairs.

I can't make very good sense of the *center* of things, what a *sequence* is, or the way shapes are placed in relationship to one another, but it is very different from the agonizing trouble I've been having for the last eight years. Now it is like having an explosion of joyful curiosity as I flail around and suck in the meaning of these concepts. Several times I have burst out laughing, reflecting that I must look like a crazy person swinging my arms around, dancing, as my body explores its new world.

On the downside I have noticed that I have begun to have some minor short-term memory problems, and pronounced trouble in retrieving nouns.

On the good side, I very distinctly notice the return of a whole *memory-scape* of symbols based on visual memories from my childhood (say ages 3–12) that make me feel connected, wise, smarter, and as though I can see the world with greater depth. Many *symbolic* memories from childhood— scenes in which I first formed the symbols I later would use for complex cognition—have become re-accessible to me. They tend to be very specific visual scenes, but are abstract in their nature, and I am now, once again, able to use them as part of the core of my representational thinking.

I also have the sense of a shadowy presence over my right shoulder about thirty feet back.

[The Ghost!]

I think of the "Quantum Symphony" device I own that does electrical line conditioning for my stereo system. It is hard to describe what this device does, but when you turn it off, all the music just gets "sad" by comparison. This is wonderfully analogous to what I experience with the glasses / return of the childhood-memory-symbols: without the glasses on, and without the increased symbolic processing ability I get with them, everything just gets *sad*. The *vibrancy* is drained away from life.

I especially notice the memories, and the "broad, deep, thinking scape" when I am listening to music. I can once again sink deeply into the space of what makes music meaningful, spiritual, and uplifting.

I also notice that there is a pie slice on my right side where cognition (the ability to conceive of, and manipulate symbols) is still fuzzy. It is better with the glasses, but still weak compared to my new, explosively vibrant left-hand side.

Ultimately I have really grown to love these glasses, and they have made phenomenal changes in my cognition, peaking in the emotional reuniting with my old self during the second week. I hate to take them off. When I remove them, within just a few minutes I start to sink back into the mire of concussion.

On February 20th, 2008, after wearing the Phase I glasses for only twelve days, I noted the following in an e-mail note to Drs. Markus and Zelinsky:

All of the following occur off and on. With periods of rest (as in no cognitive demands or brain-controlled physical demands on me), the symptoms recede. Under brain stress the symptoms become increasingly dramatic.

1. I find that I am "throwing myself around" to get from one location to another.

2. Connected with the above, my muscles are slightly (but . . . pleasantly?) cramped up so that I am hunched over when I

stand. [. . .] I don't really walk, but rather shuffle/jog/dance to get from one place to another, using my arms to help with locomotion.

3. I turn corners, or change directions, by flinging my arms in a gross hurling motion that alters my course.

4. I am experiencing an increase in the number of incidents of being unable to get through doorways, start down stairways, and so on. I have trouble "initiating" movements that have a low-level connection between shapes/lines in the real world, and being able to move toward, or through, them. I am having trouble turning *right* more often, so end up dancing around in circles to the left all the time as I navigate through the work day. All this, however, is very much *unlike* how I used to get stuck, and have trouble initiating. Then I was just bone-achingly depleted, and it sometimes took weeks to recover my energy. This, now, is more like normal fatigue because everything is so new and interesting. 'like a little kid getting worn out by bedtime.

5. I am much less able to "fake" looking normal. It is hard to disguise looking like a weirdo throwing his arms around, dancing down the hall, head and eyes shaking around. However, with mild to strong effort I can force myself to quiesce. But then as soon as I relax, my body starts off again, flailing around like a four-month-old baby playing with his environment.

   [. . .]

7. I have been more productive at work than I would have expected.

8. It is more like I am worried that I am inconveniencing others by being such an eccentric, rather than that I am suffering. In fact, in a strange way, I am celebrating being alive again.

[. . .]

11. My eyes sometimes wander around as though I am agitated, and I find myself visually examining every facet of rooms into which I have just come. I find myself vacantly "looking" at things when listening to others, though this is a function, actually, of doing nothing except attending to what they are saying.

12. Interestingly, I cannot see the *Gregory's Dalmatian** image very well with two eyes, but I see it passably with just my right, and more clearly with just my left.

I returned to Zelinsky's office on February 26th, 2008, and my brain had already changed significantly—after only two and a half weeks with the glasses. I was comfortable, and balanced, on both the right and left prism walks. My habitual position for eye aiming, as tested with Von Graefe, was now normal: in the distance I was aiming straight ahead, and up close I was just slightly outward, exactly as I was supposed to be. My plastic brain was performing its magic.

Zelinsky noted a high AC/A ratio when she put light on the center of my eyes (having to do with eye aiming), but when she used temporary lenses to change my focusing system just a little, it changed my aiming system a great deal, showing a high connectivity between the two systems. I had a hairpin trigger between my focusing and aiming systems. Zelinsky also measured a

---

*A special picture used by Richard Gregory to illustrate the top-down guiding of human cognition in vision.

cyclotorsion (a slight rotating inward of the eye when the eyes look up close and downward)—more in my right eye than in my left.

With the Phase I glasses, my Z-Bell™ Test was stable, and much improved. I was also much better at visual localization, and could now readily find the pencil eraser with my eyes closed.

Zelinsky decided that it was already time for me to move to Phase II. For the new prescription, she kept the light angled from the right with the directive yoked prisms. Then she added a bifocal reading prescription, and also a slight (but not full) nearsighted prescription to give me a little better focus on targets at a distance, correcting me to 20/30. She did nothing to help my background vision, which was now better balanced.

Zelinsky had several goals for Phase II. First, she was going for a little more comfort by giving me better focus on near and far objects. (That is, I could see better.) But she was also, at the same time, pushing me to be more flexible in being able to shift my gaze from near to far. By not emphasizing the background, she was pushing me to reorganize the surrounding space on my own, because I was now already reorienting internally. Her thinking was that because the background was more comfortable, I would be able to shift my gaze within it more easily.

I was immediately comfortable with my Phase II glasses, and they always felt well balanced, though I did miss the wild, creative left-hand space of the first pair. With these glasses, and the work I was doing with Donalee, I was rapidly progressing back toward normal life. Along the way I experienced some rather striking symptoms during the process of change. And I found that in addition to restoring cognitive abilities I had lost, the parallel treatments also started to correct attention weaknesses that had been present prior to the crash.

Several themes were dominant: In the early days of adjusting to these glasses I had mild full-body spasms wherein all my muscle groups took turns flexing, though in an almost pleasurable way—the feeling was like stretching in the morning. The contortions lasted all day long, though there was an ebb and flow to them, increasing as my brain grew fatigued under cognitive load. My knees and toes were turned inward—the left more than the right—and this left me with a strange loping pigeon-toed gait when I walked. Although I had no trouble keeping my eyes focused on objects, my head was often in constant motion, rolling around on my shoulders in all manner of odd postures. A mild version of the side-to-side seizures also appeared from time to time. At my most affected, walking down a hallway became a strange comical dance as one set of muscles flexed all together, and then another. The biggest problem was that it looked really odd—it was difficult to suppress and impossible to hide—though there was a surprising grace to my movements as I bobbed along.

After several weeks I began to experience a Zen-like calming of the inner dialogue I had been listening to in my head since my earliest memories of childhood.

The "dark" slice on my right-hand side began to open up (though not all the way), and with these Phase II glasses my hearing and ability to think in that part of my world was emphasized. Accordingly I found myself more grounded, with a tendency to be more logical and less dreamy than I was with the Phase I "left-hand-side" glasses. I was able to effortlessly turn right when I needed to. I could see the right-hand side of complex symbols, like lists and sequences, in my mind's eye. And though I tired if I had to focus too hard on the right-hand side of one of these symbolic objects, it was a *normal* tired, as though I'd had a broken arm, the cast was off, and my arm was still just a little weak.

Despite these and many other symptoms, my work was not

negatively affected, and I was becoming more productive. While sometimes startling, the changes nonetheless felt intuitively "right."

> *March 14th:* I hear more intellectual detail in music, but it is also less emotionally engaging. I hear more of the *structure* of the sound, but am getting less of the deeper thematic meaning. I also hear less of the rhythmic interplay than I did with my Phase I glasses, which rhythm I now understand is more about a pulling, tugging kind of passion.
>
> When I look at objects, especially first thing in the morning, there is a strange, rapid shaking/blurriness for a moment, and even then I do not always fully focus. The effect is like when trying to adjust one's eyes for stereoscopic photos, but it happens automatically.
>
> My reading has changed. I usually do not read particularly fast (~350 words a minute), and tend to hear the words in my head—though my reading pace is two or three times that of my speech. In the past, to speed-read—which I've several times studied recreationally—I have to work at "getting over the hump," where I just put the words in front of my eyes and see the images they generate. It always takes days of work, and I never have gotten to where it becomes automatic; I have always had to keep pushing myself.
>
> Now I notice myself almost naturally speeding through passages without the aural accompaniment of the words, as though I am simply

gracefully floating into speed-reading. Intuitively, this is connected with a lessening of the constant dialogue—chatter—in my head that has previously always attended my normal activities during the day.

March 17th–31st: I continue to be very *grounded*, and comfortable in my body. I have more energy. Today I slept later than I have in a year. I am distinctly getting more satisfaction from my dreams.

I still feel starved for calories, and am consuming large quantities of Coca-Cola and candy. But I have also lost three of the six pounds I gained last month. Am I burning up the calories in my brain?

There have been changes in my sexuality. I am (and think most males are . . .) naturally interested in the beauty of women in a very *visual* way. When Qianwei happens to be in town, I notice that I am now seeing her in a different and more sexually-enhanced way. I sense her walk, her scent, the sound of her voice, and so on, differently/better because I "see" her more clearly. I can "see" her femaleness. That is, I have a sense of her (and others) being essentially different from me in a male/female way that is one component at the heart of attraction.

April 17th: It is no coincidence that I have not updated these notes in more than two weeks. My inner dialogue has considerably slowed down. Along with the slowdown, I am much more comfortable letting things go. In this case, I have let the notes go.

What I notice is a peacefulness in all my muscles, as though I had just taken two Ibuprofen and had a glass of wine. I am able to just sit and look at people, at situations, at the world, in real time, without continually thinking about everything, and talking it over in my head. I can't ever recall such an extended period of internal quiet like this in my life.

I am also very specifically less *vigilant*. For example, when driving I am not continually checking left and right when it is not necessary to do so, such as when waiting at a red light. Instead, I'll sit calmly and look straight ahead. I am getting much more information from my peripheral vision without having to turn my head and eyes all the time. I am no longer prompted to attend to all manner of unrelated objects that grab my attention beside the road (and about which I have no interest, such as advertising billboards).*

My memory is noticeably malfunctioning, specifically for the retrieval of names. I am experiencing roughly twenty-five such memory failures a day.

I find I must be intentional about moral choices. Ordinarily there has been an inner dialogue that

---

*Zelinsky later commented that this calming was a direct result of the lessening of the activation of my fight-flight-or-fright (sympathetic) nervous system, effecting a better balance with my rest-digest (parasympathetic) nervous system.

"tells" me to do the right thing, constantly. Now that dialogue has lessened, and so I have to *choose* to be moral. I just do not care as much. It's as though I trust who I am more than I used to, and don't need to always prove it by doing the right thing.

April 26th: I continue to have a Zen-like absence of inner dialogue. I am very alert. When I need to start my mind for something, I do. I estimate that my ongoing inner dialogue is 1/5th of what it has been my whole life. There is much less use of my mind's eye for visualizing, ruminating, worrying, judging, seeing future outcomes, etc., all the time.

Qianwei is off to China for several months, so I am parenting on my own. Lucy, Paul, and Erin all needed rides, help with schoolwork, and so on this weekend, but I was still able to complete long and difficult collections of Donalee's follow-the-rule exercises each evening. I was tired afterwards, but had no breakdowns of any kind. My cognitive stamina is phenomenally improved.

On Donalee's exercises I am getting much better at figuring out the rules, following them, performing the necessary practice, and THEN moving on. In the past I would jump immediately to the solution phase, and skip the deep *process understanding* phase that comes with repetition. I do not seem to mind the intentional rote work as much because I do not have such a strong need for novel input. That is, just doing the work is satisfying in itself. I don't always need something new to distract me.

Rather than trying to "fix" chaotic social problems that arise in my environment, I just notice ("see") the bigger picture, and move on to something else, or wait quietly until others calm down. In the end this is likely to be a good thing, but it does require change in others around me. I feel increased freedom to choose my actions, and am much less driven by anxiety over what others are thinking, and anxiety about the future.*

The memory difficulties are a downside. My intuition is that I'll figure out how to start remembering things again, but without all the chaotic, vigilant refreshing of every last damn thing in my life.

I can summarize my state as "I no longer care [about the details]." But this is a positive. It was exhausting to care about everything, so now I choose not to, and I am not so worn out all the time.

On May 1st, 2008, in assessing me for my Phase III glasses, Zelinsky repeated only my eyesight tests. I had been in regular e-mail contact with her, so she already knew of the relatively dramatic cognitive changes that had been taking place.

She noted that there were three choices of action she could now take: First, she could emphasize the background again. Second, she could angle the light straight from the front (by removing the prisms), and lessen it from the right, removing the crutch I had been using in jump-starting the use of my new

---

*This preference for calm, and avoiding chaos—which affected whom I chose to spend my time with—ultimately led to quite profound changes in my life.

pathways to the visual cortex. Or, third, she could angle the light from the left, pushing me into the "bad" area, to force more adaptation to the new signal paths. She decided on the second option.

Zelinsky also added components for clarifying the target both up close in the reading prescription, and also at a distance, continuing the theme of requiring me to cover a greater range of shift in my focus. Lastly, she added a component for an astigmatism in my left eye. This last sharpens the central eyesight, but distorts the peripheral eyesight. Previously, when she had measured me in her office, I had not been able to tolerate this distortion.

So I was going to be pushed again, in several ways, and I would lose the prisms, which meant that I was now going to have to find the new brain pathways on my own.*

However, in a revealing twist of fate, a week before my Phase III glasses were shipped back from the lab, disaster struck: I lost my Phase II glasses, and made an important discovery. Despite the monumental changes the glasses were making in my life, *they did not seem to provide "residual" benefits when I wasn't wearing them.* Through a series of coincidences, I ended up, briefly, without any brain glasses at all. I regressed dramatically, and almost immediately.

> *May 6th, 2008:* I lost my Phase II brain glasses
> yesterday at 11:00 AM, at the bank, probably from
> leaving them on top of the car when I was

---

*This is a form of what contemporary brain-plasticity researcher Michael Merzenich, M.D., refers to as "use it or lose it," the principle by which the plastic brain reconfigures itself. In this case, the bad pathways had become less dominant from disuse, such that even when switching back to having light enter from the front, I should still be able to find the new pathways that had been created.

struggling to get Erin out of her car seat. I have now gone thirty-three hours without them. I no longer have access to my Phase I lenses, and my Phase III glasses will not be here until the end of the week.

I have remarkably regressed, although the "echo" of the magic glasses remains. I find myself anxious, afraid about an uncertain future. By the end of the day, and in the morning, after sleeping, I am just worn out, in the old, bad way. It is just so much work, again, to be alive.

I am starting to feel non-human again. I am sad that I can only see "locally" and have lost my global, magic, bigger-picture, overview vision. I feel disconnected from the universe and lonely.

Small tasks are harder for me to initiate (grading papers, deciding what to do today, working on Donalee's exercises). I am avoiding them because they are just "too hard."

I cannot *hear* in the same way. I cannot make sense of the sound picture in the world around me.

I am anxious, as though my eyes, and my attention, are darting around.

I am fearfully avoiding conflicts, because of my weakened state.

I cannot get "home," and I am not sure where I am.

May 7th: I continue to feel the loss of my "magic glasses."

My reading has changed back. I am hearing the words in my head as I read and this slows me down and reduces comprehension. It is less fun to read, more work.

My handwriting has regressed. It is noticeably more work to write neatly. It is as though I am in too much of a hurry, and my body is cramped up from brain to shoulder to arm to hand, making it an effort to follow through on writing out the full sweep of letters.

. . . worn out just trying to figure out what to do next . . . hard to keep doing whatever it is that I am engaged in instead of thinking about doing something else . . . have to keep a hand on the wall for balance . . . struggle to remain calm instead of anxious . . . don't look forward to tasks because they all seem to involve pain of some kind . . . my head hurts often . . . I am dreaming more about frustrating events . . . waking up early with anxiety and not going back to sleep . . .

I am inappropriately and over-vigilantly concerned about the well-being of others around me: Erin at the baby-sitter's, Qianwei in China, Paul's math, Lucy's friends, Nell's schedule, Peter all the time . . .

May 9th: I had more anxious dreams that did not resolve: my dreams are again not productive. I've lost the NSEW grid that connects them to my life.

As a scientist, I've had to allow the unlikely, but *possible* chance that my impairment and recovery were psychosomatic in nature, and that even when I lost my glasses I was simply psychosomatically re-creating the original symptoms of my so-called brain damage. However, given the steady re-onset of the original symptoms over the course of three days, and the complete lack of any psychological charge one way or the other, and the nature of the experience, this becomes ever more emphatically unlikely. And how likely is it that I could psychosomatically affect my dreams? I also had the evidence of the visually triggered seizures, which I could not reproduce on my own. Much more reasonable an explanation is that the light entering my retinas is no longer being rerouted, and visual signals are no longer traveling along the healthy pathways, thus re-triggering my brain dysfunction.

This also lays to rest the idea that my recovery was a coincidence, and I was going to spontaneously get better at this point in my life (eight years later!) on my own.

Besides the re-onset of all of the original symptoms, my over-arching experience is the stark realization of how extremely *difficult* just getting through the day has become. I am again exhausted by the simplest tasks. I have a sense of being "done for the day" before the first hour has passed.

May 9th, in the afternoon: [I had been without any brain glasses for fifty-two hours at this point.] I put on my new Phase III brain glasses, and within ten minutes have started feeling better. In an hour I am mostly back to normal. Such a short time for me to again have my vision into this alternate universe!

What a relief . . .

I feel at peace all over my body. This is not a drugged feeling, but rather just a deep quiet *normalness* with good feeling in it. My mind is quiet. I feel quietly happy. I am looking forward to the rest of my life.

Despite the bad start to the day I am now feeling physically energetic, like a rocket heading forward.

I came home from Zelinsky's and played Beatles songs on the piano (by ear) with great enthusiasm. I am distinctly less chaotic in my musical *thinking*. I also have a strong feeling of being so internally quiet that I can now better hear the joy actually present in the musical fabric itself.

These Phase III glasses, like the Phase II glasses, also emphasize the right part of my world, but the delineation lines of the magic world are significantly less well-defined. The Phase I glasses had a very distinct left pie slice. The Phase II glasses had a clear right-ish pie slice, but while these Phase III glasses are also to the right I cannot feel, or describe, the demarcation of the space very well. They are also broader from top to bottom—a wider (cognitive) vertical band.

Additionally, they feel *unbalanced* from one eye to the other, in an unsettling and challenging way:

Zelinsky has made it clear to me that she wants to make some very specific changes in my brain, and that my brain is now ready to have her make them. I suppose these Phase III glasses will achieve the results, but it is clear I am going to have to work at it.

As a professor, I recognized a rare research opportunity: given what had happened when I lost my glasses, I suggested to both Zelinsky and Markus that I stop wearing my glasses for a while, and have them take careful, possibly daily measurements and assess the changes that were taking place during my regression—sort of a temporary *Flowers for Algernon* case study. Each of them was independently aghast, considering me essentially out of my mind for being willing to take such a risk. They are, first and foremost, clinicians in the business of making individual people better, and their ethics forbid them from taking a chance with one of their patients in the interests of research, however tempted they might be as scientists. With the thought of providing what might be extremely valuable research data, I considered forcing the issue by making a unilateral decision to present the opportunity to them if they wished to record the data (that is, I would stop wearing the glasses on my own), but in the end decided I could neither go against their wishes nor take a chance with my brain because of my responsibilities as a parent. But I was tempted!*

It was very hard for me to adjust to the Phase III glasses. My intuition is that it was because of the loss of the prisms.

---

*Now, years later, I find that my brain has rewired itself through habituation, and I am not nearly so dependent on my glasses.

Wearing the new glasses was unsettling, and with them I felt a change in my personality. From my notes:

> *May 22nd, 2008:* I find myself dreamier in very specific ways. It is harder for me to attend to narratives when people are talking. It is not so much that I drift off, but rather that I pay attention to other parts of them—who they are, what they look like, and sound like—rather than just what they are saying.
>
> I am more annoyed by noises such as lawnmowers, refrigerators, a noisy computer fan . . . I have less sense of my left and right magical hearing spaces . . .
>
> I got into minor social tussles with two difficult people. I was clearly in the right in both cases, and also very reasonable. However, I noticed that I was more reactive, and concerned about "fairness," than I would have been with the Phase II glasses. Wearing those I would have been calmer, and would have just patiently listened to the unfair things being said, without responding. While the issues were each resolved quickly, and amicably, I was disappointed: first that the tussles occurred at all, and second, that I was bothered about it when they did.
>
> My handwriting has deteriorated again. While it is *possible* for me to force myself to write neatly, as with the Phase II glasses, it is not natural. I am again dropping pieces of individual letters, taking shortcuts in my cursive writing. I am in a hurry

when I write, and my muscles aren't working in the same way.

I am quite productive. I've gotten much done this week. I've been able to prioritize, and then calmly choose victim tasks that I won't be able to get to, without worrying about them. I have a strong sense of intentionality and choice.

May 29th: I've experienced a natural and striking increase in my ability to find keys on the piano and to play simple pieces by ear in twelve different keys. It is significantly easier for me to "see" the notes in relation to one another as I pick out tunes, counterpoint, and chords. I am more easily absorbing the visual patterns of the keys, and the sounds are more accurately linked to those patterns.

Because I could see better with the Phase III glasses, I tended to wear them at night while driving.

From the beginning I found the Phase III glasses "unbalanced," as though one eye was seeing the world differently from the other. Each time I changed my focus from near to far, or vice versa, there was a lag before my eyes agreed on what they were seeing.

I picked up my Phase II replacement glasses on May 27th. They were immediately more comfortable, and because there were so many end-of-the-school-year demands on me, I mostly went back to wearing them, though I still wore my Phase III glasses when driving at night. I sent a note to Zelinsky explaining, but she verified that this was the correct prescription. She suggested that I continue to trade off between the two pairs until I could make the transition. I had work to do. The timetable was up to me.

In late June 2008 I began a regimen of wearing the Phase III glasses a few hours a day, and the Phase II glasses the rest of the time. This lasted for more than a year. Then, during an extended August 2009 working vacation at my mother's rural property in northern California, where the demands on me were lessened, I put the Phase II glasses away and forced myself to wear the Phase III glasses for long periods each day.

> *August 26th, 2009:* During this whole month past the Phase III glasses have continued to feel "unbalanced." I have to work hard at wearing them. Over time, however, I have grown to tolerate them. When I tried going back to my Phase II glasses a few days ago I found that it was like regressing from being a responsible adult back into some sort of adolescence: although it has been painful to move on to a more profound state of recovery, I no longer find it attractive to go back. Time to grow up!

After that month in California I was able to wear the Phase III glasses all the time for several months. I was never comfortable with them and how they presented the external world to me, but I *was* happy with what they did for me internally. My cognition was again further improved.

Zelinsky later explained to me that my lopsided feeling was because, in fact, the targets in the two eyes *were* sharpened in different ways. One was magnified slightly more than was the other, intentionally forcing my brain to readjust the balance between one eye and the other every time I changed the near/far focus of my gaze.

On October 15th, 2009, after fifteen months with the Phase III glasses, I returned to the Mind-Eye Connection and was tested for my Phase IV glasses.

From 10:15 until 11:00 A.M., I went through preliminary review and testing with Martha. I filled her in on some of the observations I'd been making in my diary. "On the good side," I said, "I experience a general state of joy, peacefulness, and calm well-being. I feel much less need for vigilance. I have more choice in what I attend to. My house is significantly more ordered.

"On maybe the bad side, but also maybe still good, I'll report two strange things: First, the *quality* of my listening to people is different. When people are talking to me about themselves, I am noticeably less interested in the story—that is, the 'drama'—and in the context. Instead I find myself paying close attention to the person speaking, and the qualities of *who they are* as they speak. But I am no longer *compelled* to *become the story with them.*

"This might be bad in that I am just a less compassionate person. It might be good in that I can choose to be compassionate, but am not driven to be. I have more choice. It might be good that I'm attending more to the actual people, and their immediate experiences, than to the stories they are telling, which might even be a better form of compassion."

Martha listened carefully to what I was saying, and wrote it down. I went on: "Second, I am less responsive to appropriate stress which is, correctly, prompting me to get some job done—I just don't care as much and am more accepting of possible negative consequences."

Martha, who seemed to have heard this before from other

patients, asked, "Is it like this: People are coming over, and you get your whole house in order, except that you don't get the front hall cleaned? You just don't quite get to everything, but you don't worry about it and enjoy your guests anyway?"

"Yes!" I said. "That's right."

Then I extended the example. "Actually, it's more like the *first* time they come over the front hall isn't clean, and that's not so great. But my head is less cluttered with things I'm worried about. I have a little bit more time and energy each day, and, as a consequence, over time, I have more time to *keep* my house clean. In a few months, I am not only not stressed about every last thing, but my house is also already clean when guests come over. I can't count on myself to achieve every last goal anymore, but in the end I seem to be coming out ahead."

Martha continued to write everything down. It was all data to Zelinsky, and also to her then-associate, Lisa Kowar, O.D. How gratifying it was to have people note the actual details of my experience before deciding how to proceed!

Martha then completed my testing with the Padula Visual Midline Shift test, the H-pursuit test, the Visual Localization Test, and so on.

From 11:00 A.M. until noon I saw the wonderful Dr. Kowar, who carefully reviewed Martha's notes and then performed her own extensive testing with the phoropter, with single-eye occlusions, with eye charts, and so on. She focused extensively on my binocular vision, and on fixation disparity. We tried many different lenses. She wrote up her results and passed these on to Zelinsky.

From noon until 12:45 P.M. I met with Zelinsky in her examination room.

In looking over the tests that Martha had performed, and the notes she had taken, Zelinsky said, "You're doing very well.

Your brain has changed. It's adjusting." She referred to my feelings of contentment and peace. "However, you're no longer performing optimally on the Z-Bell Test, or on the Von Graefe Phoria Test."

She reviewed Dr. Kowar's notes, and performed a Z-Bell™ Test with the lenses that Dr. Kowar recommended. She said, "Dr. Kowar got this just right. She's right on."

But still she wasn't satisfied. She tried different lenses and repeated the Z-Bell™ Test, and one of the fixation disparity tests. Then she and Dr. Kowar started a long conversation that lasted, off and on, for the next hour. The issue was to make a decision about how much stress to put me under in making further changes. They could make me more comfortable with the prescription, but then would possibly lose an opportunity to push me farther along the path they wanted my plastic brain to travel.

Dr. Kowar decided to retest me with a portable handheld lens apparatus. It was less convenient than the phoropter, but in my case important, because it removed some of the phoropter's blocking of peripheral, nonvisual retinal signals from the testing equation. So I spent another half hour with her, from 1:45 until 2:15 P.M.

Our dialogue is revealing of the detailed work that went into determining the final prescription. This may sound like something out of a séance, but in fact, it shows the extreme sensitivity I had developed to my nonvisual retinal processing (possibly enhanced by my years of "moving energy around" with my Tai Chi practice?), and also illustrates Dr. Kowar's long experience in teasing out necessary information from her patients.

Dr. Kowar put together the handheld versions of the recommended lenses, and then ran me through the Z-Bell™ Test. "Ah-HAH!" she said triumphantly. "I THOUGHT so!" With the handhelds I now measured incorrectly on both sides. She made slight adjustments, and asked me, "How's that?"

Me: "Okay, I guess. My hearing/symbol space is tilted diagonally up on the right side, and definitely emphasizes the right side over the left. But it's all right."

Kowar (laughing): "Well, we don't want you to be lopsided . . ."

She tried a different configuration. "Now?"

Me: "The diagonal has flattened out a little, closer now to being horizontal."

Kowar (after more changes): "How about now?"

Me: "That opens everything up on the left side. A little narrower cognitive space on the right side. I can't think quite as well over there now."

Kowar: "How is the diagonal? Are you still tipped?"

Me: "No, that seems to have leveled out. I'm very comfortable."

Kowar tried the Z-Bells again, checking. I nailed them right on center each time, but even so, she tried a slightly different lens on the left side again. "How about now?"

Me: "It's okay, but I'm not quite comfortable."

Kowar: "Oh. How?"

Me: "Well, it's a little hard to describe, but it's as though I'm nervous, or unsettled."

. . . and so on for the next half hour.

Dr. Kowar could have gotten all of the same information by taking measurements on my response lag to near and far focus, looking at my altered fixation disparity, and so on, in addition to using the Z-Bell™ Test, as we tried different lenses. But, because of my sensitivity, the self-reporting dialogue was more efficient.

To get a feel for the "symbolic working space" we discussed, try the following: Close your eyes and picture, up close, the detailed process of tying the bowknot in a pair of lace-up shoes. As you tie it—in your mind's eye—describe the scene out loud. (This places a verbal-translation load on your brain, in addition to the visualization load.) Push yourself to actually follow all of the bends and twists in each half of the lace. Now repeat the exercise, all the way through, in eight different spots—upper left three feet away, middle far right one foot away, and so on. Can you see the process clearly in each location? Are you comfortable in each part of your symbolic visual field? Most of us will have preferred work areas in the space around us, and some will have zones that are altogether "dead."

Drs. Kowar and Zelinsky talked over Dr. Kowar's last round of tests. With the lenses they settled on, my visual "working space" was very clear in all quadrants, and just shy of the full 180 degrees wide, stretching from perpendicular outward near my left temple to the perpendicular near my right temple. The new space was also still tilted slightly up to the right, and down to the left. I was, as Dr. Kowar had joked, "slightly lopsided." Neither Zelinsky nor Kowar had been happy with the tilting, but this was the only prescription that gave me the wide perspective, so we decided to live with it. Importantly, Zelinsky wanted to alter the way my visual target and visual background were balanced. She decided to push me to navigate and deal with space better by backing away from clarity in the prescription—in particular in my left eye (where I had the astigmatism)—and she made some other, minor changes as well. I believe that some aspect of this backing away from clarity in the center-focus prescription contributed to the sense of "mental fuzziness" I later experienced with these glasses.

This working space engendered by the Phase IV glasses was a marked change from my Phase III glasses, which, while less focused than my Phase II glasses, still clearly emphasized the right hand side of my visual plane. With the new prescription it was a pleasure to get back the full use of the creative, left-hand side of my symbolic, spatial sense as well.

> *October 22nd, 2009:* I got my Phase IV glasses today. They are immediately comfortable and do not have the challenging feel of the Phase III glasses.

> *February 5th, 2011*: [Sixteen months later] These glasses continue to be very down-to-earth. I feel a peace with them that is from being *in* the world, rather than a peace engendered by escaping from it. I am also slightly fuzzy, and a little dull.

> *June 3rd, 2011*: The Phase IV glasses have always been comfortable enough, but over the course of twenty months I have noticed that my thinking has been—or has grown—"fuzzy," as though I were getting old. It is always five o'clock on a hot day in August, and I'm looking out from a room with dirty windows. I have also noticed that the

area on my right-hand side is particularly "fuzzy" in an exteroceptive way, and that my hearing in the same quadrant is diminished and not sharply defined. I've also lost my "killer instinct" for taking on, and completing jobs.

On June 20th, 2011, I returned to Zelinsky to be assessed for my Phase V glasses. Things were going well, but I complained to her of my ongoing concern that I was "mentally fuzzy," in particular in the right side of my vision. I could not "think" in that part of my space very well, could not form mental symbols well in the area about forty-five degrees to my right and front, even though that part of my world was still being emphasized.

On most of the tests I was close to normal. Interestingly, my right eye no longer needed as strong a prescription to see clearly. (That is, my actual eyesight had improved.)

Consistent with the intuition I had expressed in my diary, Zelinsky changed the focusing balance between my eyes by decreasing the prescription strength in my right eye, and increasing it in my left eye, along with a change in the axis value. My mental fuzziness immediately cleared up, and the right-hand side of my world became clearer and more concrete. This is an interesting result, because while my right-side *vision* got less clear, I was *seeing* better, mentally, on that side, presumably because I was better emphasizing the *context* in which my target vision was unfolding.

On June 9th, 2012, a year later, I returned for another checkup, and to see about getting my Phase VI glasses. My chief complaint was that although the right-hand side of my thinking space was clear with the Phase V glasses, it was still not "vibrant." It was not *alive* in the way I would like it to be for solving hard academic problems, and, more generally, for experiencing enthusiasm in life, and for finding humor, and novelty, in the world. This may sound like a pretty esoteric complaint, but by that point I had come to know my cognitive space quite well.

Zelinsky said, "Tell me a little bit more about what you are after."

I said, "I'm productive at work. I feel peaceful. I can reason fine in both hemispheres. I'm not at all fuzzy the way I was before. Nonetheless, there is a sixty-degree pie slice *here* [I held up my hands to the right side of my head, demonstrating], from the perpendicular leaving my right temple and extending forward, that is not too *lively* compared to the rest of the space forward of it, and to the left."

Zelinsky asked, "Do you feel like you're missing a *vibrancy* or *creativity* in that pie slice? Do you particularly notice it when you're working on complex problems?"

"Yes!" I said. She was putting the right words in my mouth to describe it.

Zelinsky ran through all of her standard vision tests on the phoropter, and then finished tweaking the prescription she already had in mind with the Z-Bell™ Test. She focused only on the high bell in my upper *left* quadrant. She had a plan and knew what she was looking for. In a cursory way, she checked the upper right quadrant with the high bell, but this was right on—as she had expected—and she wasn't further interested in it.*

She then ran me through the Visual Localization Test ("Look at the eraser on the end of this pencil. Close your eyes.

---

*Over the years of working with Zelinsky I found this to be a common experience: that she often made complex predictions about what she was going to later find with her instruments. So many times I heard her say, "Now watch what happens when we . . ." and she was then proven exactly right in her prediction.

Reach out and touch the eraser") quite a few times with slightly different prescriptions before making her final decision.

Zelinsky found that by inserting small vertical directive yoked prisms (thick part on the bottom) into the lenses, and making some other small changes, she was able to perfectly increase my right-side awareness. The prescription also tilted my posture slightly backward (posture angle affects the central nervous system), and thus made me more comfortable.

When I got my Phase VI glasses back from the lab a week later, they immediately added back that spark I had been lacking with the Phase V glasses. This was the final tweak. It is these same glasses that I continue to wear today.

Donalee Markus's plan and Deborah Zelinsky's plan for me were now both complete. I was balanced, had clear logical thinking, was able to create mental images with clarity, and could feel that coveted mental vibrancy in all areas of my thinking. I felt *normal*.

My experience at the Mind-Eye Connection was far from unique. Dr. Deborah Zelinsky cares deeply about the well-being of the people she sees. She believes that the research data she has collected, the clinical case notes she has kept, and the continually refined techniques she uses can help thousands of people to lead better, happier, more productive lives. She has worked unceasingly for years because she is passionate about the work she does with her patients, and also about the vast potential for neuro-optometric rehabilitation in general. And, too, there is the constant battle in her own schedule to make time for her research when there are people who so often desperately need her help as a clinician. Like Dr. Donalee Markus, she is one of the heroes working on the leading edge of modern brain plasticity clinical research.

EPILOGUE

Wabash Avenue

As I write these closing paragraphs, I am, except in a few small ways, free from concussion symptoms. I can focus on complex problems again without pain or nausea. I can work for long periods of time. I can multitask, within reason. I can again say prayers and meditate. My balance problems are not significant. My sense of direction has returned, and I can make decisions without difficulty. And, too, because I have addressed dispositional attention difficulties as part of my treatment, many areas of my life have even improved over how I was prior to the crash: my house, my life, and my relationships are significantly less chaotic because I *see* my choices more clearly.

As I think back to how far I've come, I recall a concussion scene from winter quarter, late at night, after teaching an evening class at DePaul.

I had been sitting in my eleventh-floor Lewis Center classroom for an hour after class, staring at the wall. Now, I had trouble getting through the doorway, and also had to hold on to the wall to make it to the elevator foyer. Taking the elevators to the first floor would leave me unable to walk, or to stand, and I felt I couldn't risk making a scene with the security guard. So I took the stairs, holding on to railings the whole way down, and guiding myself step-by-step along the wall. Several times I had to crawl, and several times I got stuck, unable to move at all.

About forty minutes later I left the building through the Jackson Street doors—headed for my office in a building on the next street. I was moving in slow motion, holding on to the building's outer wall for balance.

The tracks for the Chicago El train ran along Wabash Avenue, and I had to pass under them when I crossed Wabash on the way back to my office. Several lines ran on those tracks, and trains also came around the turn at Van Buren to the south, so it was not always possible to know exactly when the trains were coming, or when a hidden train, stopped just a block north at the Adams station, might start up and head south over the Jackson intersection.

Because the tracks were perched on steel pillars (that is, you could look up and see the sky through the tracks), the sound of the trains could be very loud. The wheels sometimes emitted a loud squeal as the trains made their way down the tracks or came around the bend. If this caught me off guard, I would clap my hands over my ears and double over—the same as I did with Ramon's disc brakes. Sometimes I would fall to the ground holding my head. As long as I was on the sidewalk this was merely embarrassing, but otherwise not so much trouble. On this evening, however, I miscalculated, and was under the tracks, in the middle of Wabash Avenue, when a squealing train came by. I felt an explosion go off in my head as I fell to the salty, wet pavement, and curled up on the street in fetal position, covering my ears.

The train passed, but my mind and body were moving in slow motion. Before I could get up, the traffic light changed. Cars traveling down the one-way slalom on Wabash—avoiding the steel support pillars for the El—started swerving past me on both sides, in the dark, their horns blaring only a few feet away from my head. Each time they did so, with their headlights also blinding me as they passed, another cognitive explosion went off, flooding me with a brain-piercing stream of unfiltered sensory information. Other cars came around the corner, making the turn south from Jackson. Startled, their drivers too honked impatiently as they rushed past.

It was a bizarre fantasy sequence out of a Hollywood nightmare scene—except that it was real.

But this had happened to me before. I thought that at some point the traffic would clear and I would make it to the far sidewalk. I would prop myself up next to the streetlight, hope that no one I knew was around at that late hour, and then go about the rest of my much-altered life.

Yet even then, amid the chaos of my life—but also within the larger mystery of compassion that can ever reach back and find us—the Ghost was there perched in the distance, still tethered to me by the merest thread of possibility, waiting for the miracle.

I dedicate this book to you, Dr. Donalee Markus, and to you, Dr. Deborah Zelinsky. Thank you for coming to get us.

APPENDIX

DOTS PUZZLES

Find all instances of the appropriate three shapes in each of the following two puzzles. Every dot will be used.

2D PAGE OF DOTS OVERLAID

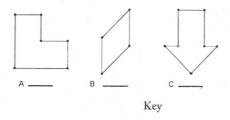

Key

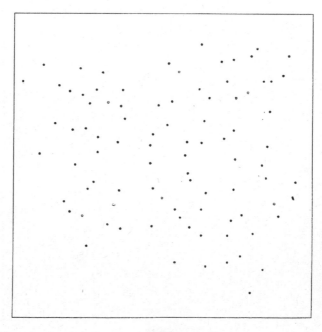

Puzzle

3D PAGE OF DOTS OVERLAID

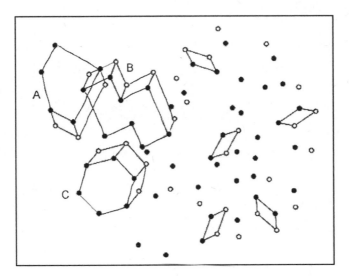

Key

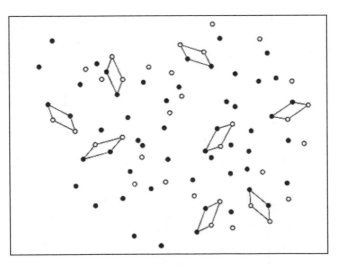

Puzzle

ACKNOWLEDGMENTS

I would like to thank the following people who were essential in bringing this manuscript to life. In chronological order: Donalee Markus, and Deborah Zelinsky, who agreed to painstakingly verify all of the notes on my recovery; my good friend the writer Pamela Janis, the catalyst who turned a collection of notes into a real book and has been the best champion for it from the start; Leslie Breed, who graciously gave her time early in this project; Howard Yoon, whose reputation as one of the finest agents in the business does not do justice to the breadth of his kindness and compassion as a human being; Melanie Tortoroli, who blessed us with her essential editing gifts and global patience in managing so many aspects of this large project; my daughter Nell Elliott, whose insight and skill are everywhere present through the six thousand edits she made in the manuscript, and the structural design she suggested; our copy editor, Michael Burke, who painstakingly cleaned up the text throughout with the logic and precision of

ACKNOWLEDGMENTS

a scientist; Georgia Bodnar, who managed all the art; and all of the other professionals at Viking who tolerated me as an academic used to fighting over every comma. I'd especially like to thank all of those in the DePaul community who were so supportive, including, but not limited to, my compassionate deans Helmut Epp, and David Miller, and my colleagues Gary Andrus, Adam Steele, and Greg Brewster.

INDEX